MAXIMUM FITNESS
FITNESS
Minimum
Risk

MAXIMUM FITNESS
Minimum Risk

**The Wellness Exercise Program
for Cardiac, Diabetes, and
Pulmonary Patients**

CAROLE MARSHALL

CAVEAT PRESS
Ashland, Oregon

Inquiries should be addressed to:
Caveat Press
PO Box 3400
Ashland, Oregon 97520
www.caveatpress.com

Printed in the United States of America

First printing: 2005

Cover by Lightbourne Design, Inc.
Interior by Christy Collins

Library of Congress Cataloging-in-Publication Data

Marshall, Carole.
    Maximum fitness—minimum risk : the wellness exercise program for cardiac, diabetes, and pulmonary patients / by Carole Marshall.
        p. cm.
    Includes bibliographical references.
    ISBN 0-9745245-0-6 (pbk.)
    1. Chronic diseases--Exercise therapy. 2. Physical fitness. 3. Health promotion. 4. Hospitals--Health promotion services. I. Title.

RC108.M37 2004
616.1'062--dc22

                                    2004019410

The ideas, exercises, and suggestions contained in this book are intended to help you benefit from a supervised program in a hospital setting. This book is not a substitute for appropriate advice from your healthcare provider for your specific medical condition.

TABLE OF CONTENTS

PREFACE

MAXIMUM FITNESS-MINIMUM RISK defines an optimal health opportunity for cardiac, diabetes, and pulmonary clients in the safe, medically supervised setting of a hospital affiliated wellness facility. It is a guide through the three phases of a basic wellness program with an emphasis on exercise. The intention of this book is to create awareness and decrease intimidation and confusion. It is an invitation for you to begin a wellness adventure.

The hospital wellness program has a community-oriented curriculum that encompasses a wide variety of outpatient needs. One segment of the wellness agenda provides education, exercise, and support to chronically ill clients. This can include one-on-one counseling, educational classes specific to illness, and individually designed exercise prescriptions.

No two wellness programs are the same. Days and times of operation vary. Structures are different. The maintenance phase, as defined, may not be available. Some wellness Phase II diabetes programs are educational only. In addition, exercise equipment is not exact to every gym, and exercise sessions are documented differently from program to program. Facilities may use computers, personal charts, individual workout logs, or a combination of documentations. The variations as well as the similarities are many, but the absolute commonality is the dedication of staff and the grit of participants.

During my years as a wellness personal trainer, I was privy to every aspect of this program and hold in high regard the dedicated personnel and determined clients. With my focus on exercise, I have had the joy and privilege of helping people work toward improved fitness and functional independence through the experience of safe exercise.

Getting involved in a workout routine with a diagnosis of heart disease, diabetes, or pulmonary problems can raise many questions and concerns. Understanding the nuts and bolts of a hospital wellness exercise program is a good way to get queries answered and put fears to rest. This project is deeply rooted in my personal goal to give back to a community that has given much to me. I have been spiritually guided every step of the way. It is my hope that all readers become informed and inspired and take the necessary steps to personal wellness.

INTRODUCTION

I REMEMBER THE DENIAL. Voices spoke of someone else as I held my eyes away from inquiring faces and separated myself from the world around me. Mourning the loss of an ordinary yesterday, I feared the unknown of a thousand tomorrows.

I remember the anger. The jolt to the soul of my personal well-being had not been part of the plan, and I despised the unsolicited change in a well-designed existence. Normal lives flourished around me, and I railed against recovery until the thickening barnacles of resentment became more harmful than the event.

I remember acceptance. It was a decision a long time in coming, but once signed on, I changed. Stronger, clearer, more focused than I had ever been, I took on the responsibility of the hand I was dealt with a willingness to seek healthy avenues of contribution and self-improvement.

My experience was the loss of a loved one, but trials come in many forms, from saying goodbye to someone dear to relinquishing good health to an unexpected illness. No one is immune to misfortune, but no matter what life gives or takes away, we always own the power of choice. My circumstance has led me to choose to use writing as a means of adding to the health and well-being of the community.

The process of moving through life is a journey of planned and unplanned events. Twists and turns along our paths are marked by pleasures and perils, joys and sorrows, ups and downs. Facing personal illness is a common and often debilitating event. As the "forever" concept of youthful stamina and buoyancy slowly wanes, the decline of health can carry a heavy weight, making physical soundness and equilibrium more elusive. A wide range of emotions manifest after the shock of a disturbing diagnosis. As I experienced with my loss, feelings of denial and anger can grip the psyche like a squeezing vice. A diagnosis of chronic illness also brings the distress of giving something up, as well as the fear of tackling an unknown. Taking time to digest the turmoil is healthy. Feelings need recognition, expression, and acknowledgement, but in order to successfully manage illness it is vitally important to traverse through the haze of disbelief and make clear, positive life choices. In *Lifetime Fitness and Wellness,* Melvin H. Williams writes, "The ultimate key to a Positive Health Life-style is an attitude of self-responsibility for your own health status."

There is an art to gracious aging. It involves deciding to make the most of life no matter the glitches, choosing to be pleasant no matter the terrain, and fostering the highest possible spiritual and physical health. "All the hardships that come to you in life, all the tribulations and nightmares, all the things you see as punishments from God are in reality like gifts. They are an opportunity to grow, which is the sole purpose of life," writes Elisabeth Kübler-Ross in *The Wheel of Life.* Chronic illness is an opportunity. Progressing with enthusiasm, interest, and dedication into the core of the issue is a way to make the best of what appears to be the worst cir- cumstance. Self-care is your choice. It involves getting on a path to personal wellness.

"Increasingly, Americans are striving toward the state of opti- mal health known as wellness," writes Dianne Hales in *An Invita- tion to Health.* Optimal, defined as most favorable or desirable, is the operative word in understanding that a state of wellness can be everyone's goal. A most favorable state of health is an individ- ual achievement. A diagnosis of diabetes, lung problems, or heart disease does not take you out of the running for optimal health. Instead, it invites exploration into the highest state of wellness possible for the conditions at hand. A necessary component for realizing a personal best fitness condition is exercise. A fitness program can be designed to afford you, as a diabetes, pulmonary, or cardiac patient, the best possible state of health, and you'll move easily into the process. No matter the pre-diagnosis exercise savvy or lack of fitness know-how of wellness clients, everyone starts at the beginning.

A diagnosis of diabetes, heart disease, or lung problems requires developing a "new normal" for quality of life. Exercise is a necessary component. Use this book to acquaint yourself with the safe, medically managed wellness exercise program that accommodates your health issue. It is your guide to action in adversity.

"If your ship doesn't come in, swim out to it."—Jonathan Winters

To wellness clients … past, present, future

1

THE DIAGNOSIS

THE AIR IS HEAVY. The sensation of pins and needles turns to a creeping numbness moving over your body like a low fog blanketing a tranquil bay. Palms sweat, your heart pounds. The urge to flee the suffocating room is overpowering. Voices become distorted echoes as the psyche refuses the diagnosis and grasps for the lost reins of independence. Your mind reaches back before the "outing" of the illness to yesterday and life as usual, back to the recall of innocence when this was someone else's disease. "I was quite surprised to be told that my aortic valve would have to be replaced," says Dick, a heart patient, "but my attitude was and continues to be if there is a medical problem that is fixable or manageable let's do it and get on with life."

Anyone who experiences a cardiac event or is diagnosed with diabetes or pulmonary disease has a lot of company. Seventeen million people in the United States have diabetes. More than sixty-one million Americans have some form of cardiovascular (heart) disease, and it is estimated that well over twenty-two million U.S. adults have evidence of diminished lung function. The most common adult respiratory problems are asthma, emphysema, and bronchitis. These conditions are grouped as chronic obstructive pulmonary disease (COPD). In part, the large numbers are due to advances in heart and diabetes care and the use of home oxygen, all of which allow patients with chronic illness to live longer today than ever before. There is also an increase in newly diagnosed cases each year in part due to out-of-control obesity, a contributing factor in diabetes, heart disease, and COPD. Sixty-four percent of Americans are overweight.

The numbers are sky-high, but joining the ranks of millions offers little consolation in the wake of a full-force hit to personal well-being. When your life is interrupted by an unexpected illness, the loss of health generates emotional upheaval. At first there's denial. "I kept telling myself it was gas so I wouldn't have to tell myself it was my heart," says a fifty-eight-year-old cardiac patient. For some, not remembering the diagnosis at all is the temporary fix, a pristine moment when rousing from the haze of sleep masks the reality. "I'd wake up and not even think about checking my blood sugar," admits a diabetes patient. "It was a whole change of routine, and I wasn't prepared for it." It's easy to forget. You feed the cat, read the newspaper, hum to an old tune playing on the radio, and life is as it was; engrossed in a favorite television show, challenging crossword puzzle, or an endless to-do list, the memory slips. The familiar rotes of business as usual sabotage the facts and put the diagnosis on the periphery, until you remember, and when you do the disbelief is devastating. Afraid and confused, you vacillate between skepticism and beating yourself up for having ignored ambiguous symptoms and procrastinated about changing unhealthy habits. "From why me to anger, patients can go through all the stages of a death experience, and what patients fear most is a loss of independence," says Dr. Sandra Smith-Poling. "Even if they haven't gone skiing in ten years, the thought that they may never do that again is devastating. A diagnosis of a chronic illness can feel like the death of independence."

As difficult as it may seem early on, acceptance will move you in the right direction, but there's an important component to keep in mind. Says Smith-Poling, "What you want from patients with a chronic illness diagnosis is acceptance with a desire to do the maximum they can to improve themselves to their maximum ability." For the best long-term results, patients must be pro-active in the management of their disease. "This should be your new job," advises Smith-Poling. Become educated and informed about your illness. Read, go to the Internet or to the library, and have friends and family bring you information pertinent to your condition. Write down questions for your doctors so you are well-prepared for medical appointments. Attend educational events and seminars relative to your illness. Learn everything you can about helping yourself. The more you know the better equipped you will be to partner with your healthcare providers in the management of your disease. "Learn the control you have over your illness," adds Smith-Poling. "When you're proactive, positive things generate more positives."

Whether working closely with your primary care physician or a specialist, *you* are the one who will have to make lifestyle changes. For the heart patient these changes will likely include the introduction of several new medications, dietary adjustments to lower sugar and fat intake, weight loss if you're obese, monitoring blood pressure and pulse rate, adding a cardiologist to your list of doctors, and yearly treadmill testing.

A diagnosis of COPD may mean using inhalers, dealing with a portable

YOUR NEW JOB

Educate yourself about your diagnosis. Get information from the Internet or library. Encourage info from family, friends, and the medical community. Attend events and seminars.

oxygen tank, prioritizing activities, managing shortness of breath, and losing weight if you're obese. You'll add respiratory specialists to your list of doctors, and have periodic pulmonary function tests.

For a diabetes diagnosis oral medications or administering insulin injections may be involved. Dietary changes will include becoming aware of carbohydrates and sugars in foods, adjusting when, what and how much you eat, always carrying a healthy snack to stabilize blood sugar, and weight loss if you're obese. Daily finger pricks to check blood glucose levels may be necessary, and you'll add a diabetes educator and dietitian to your list of medical consultants.

As overwhelming as all of this might seem, regaining control and finding a "new normal" is possible. Diabetes client Harriet says her diagnosis had a positive affect. "My feelings were rather ones of relief to find out why I was feeling so rotten and then knowing something could be done to alleviate the feeling." In *Fitness and Health*, Brian J. Sharkey, PhD, writes, "The stages of life provide many challenges and opportunities. We need an arsenal of activities and coping strategies to help us through the lows as we regain confidence and establish new goals." Finding a wealth of activities and strategies in the light of your diagnosis is an important step toward regaining confidence, and you have already begun. You've survived the blow. You are acknowledging your feelings. "What I hate most is going out in public with an oxygen tank," says a newly diagnosed pulmonary patient, "but I'm getting used to it. I can't be stuck in the house forever."

You are also gaining knowledge by gathering the information that will help reduce anxiety, and you're adapting to drug and dietary changes. In addition, you are working closely with your physician in the day-to-day supervision of your illness, but ultimately you are responsible for your health. Today, the average doctor spends only twelve minutes with a chronically ill patient. A crucial next step is devising a long-term plan for optimal health. An established support system specific to your needs can be your strongest ally as you begin this gallant journey. A wellness program is one such support system that offers its clients education, fitness instruction, on-going exercise, a trained and educated staff, and the camaraderie of motivated people who share similar experiences.

"The best thing you can do is get with people who have been successful. They are the mentors and role models," says Smith-Poling. "The community of a wellness program fosters this mentoring process." And for cardiac, diabetes, and COPD patients who participate in a wellness program, triumphs can be expected.

After years of heavy smoking, Bill—a COPD wellness client—admits he was somewhat depressed, but not too surprised when diagnosed with lung disease. "Exercise and education were a big help in managing my illness," he says. From staff to clients, the wellness family is united in the spirit of positive progress toward the highest standard of health possible. For Harriet, who did regular balance exercises at home, joining wellness exercise was an outgrowth of a diabetes education program. "I took advantage of this offer and found that the additional exercise appeared to help in the control of the sugar levels and, besides, it was enjoyable. The wellness program offered an opportunity to exercise regardless of weather and in good company."

2

THE NEXT STEP—
THE WELLNESS PROGRAM

MERRIAM WEBSTER'S COLLEGIATE DICTIONARY defines wellness as, "the quality or state of being in good health, especially as an actively sought goal." Having heart disease, diabetes, or lung problems does not take you out of the running for achieving a state of good health. In fact, some people find themselves in better shape after the diagnosis. The blinders come off, habits are evaluated, new behaviors are established, and the desire for improved quality of life sets the wheels in motion. For many, good health does become an actively sought goal, but achieving it in a sound and reasonable manner means keeping a healthy focus on your illness. A wellness program is designed to promote the highest possible conditioning while working with the intricacies of your illness. It is one of the best support systems available to the cardiac, diabetes, and COPD patient.

There are many outstanding programs that fall under the umbrella of wellness. Some offer health screenings, dietary information, handouts, patient group meetings, and access to referral services. There are facilities countrywide that provide physical and occupational therapy treatments and the countless private practices of medical, dental, vision, chiropractic, homeopathic, and counseling professionals who devote their working lives to the enrichment of your state of health. In addition, communities host wellness seminars featuring doctors, nurses, therapists, and other health educators and caregivers well-versed in chronic illness and up-to-the-minute advances and treatments. Health clubs have trainers who run wellness workout classes for senior citizens, and companies are developing employee wellness programs to initiate positive health changes. But for you as a heart, diabetes, or COPD patient, your wellness program needs to offer a combination of medically advocated education courses, individually developed and monitored workout routines, and on-going supervised exercise maintenance classes. This program, while not necessarily physically connected to a hospital, is affiliated with a medical facility. It is "incident to" physician services. "It is a program of many facets," says hospital Wellness Director Nancy Schmidt, whose long-held interest in cardiac care accelerated after her mother's untimely death from a heart attack. "From secondary prevention, community outreach and education, and employee health, to seated and table massage, support for various chronic illnesses, bereavement issues, and social contact for isolated senior citizens our goal is to stimulate clients, hospital personnel, and local citizens to actively pursue a state of wellness."

This book models the three phase hospital-affiliated wellness program for cardiac, diabetes, and COPD patients, with a specific focus on exercise. Every hospital wellness program is distinct in days and times of operation and in fitness components provided. In order to include the broad range of possible activities, the format of assigned, one-hour classes held three times per week is the schedule presented.

Highly trained medical and fitness professionals staff the wellness program recommended for clients with your illness. In *Guidelines for Cardiac Rehabilitation and Secondary Prevention Programs, Third Edition*, the American Association of Cardiovascular & Pulmonary Rehabilitation lists the following as program director minimum qualifications:

Bachelor's degree in an allied health field, such as exercise physiology, or licensure in the jurisdiction, for example, as a registered nurse or physical therapist.

Advanced knowledge of exercise physiology, nutrition, risk-factor modification strategies, counseling techniques, and uses of education programs and technologies as applied to cardiovascular rehabilitation and secondary prevention services.

Experience in staff coordination and delivery of secondary prevention services to patients.

Successful completion of Basic Life Support (BLS) or Advanced Cardiac Life Support (ACLS) (if eligible to provide such services) courses.

Certification, experience, and training equivalent to those specified for an Exercise Specialist™ by the ACSM, certification through the American Nurses Credentialing Center (ANCC), or the advance specialty in cardiopulmonary rehabilitation of the American Physical Therapy Association (APTA).

In addition to the program director, all coordinators are skilled in Advanced Cardiac Life Support (ACLS). ACLS is the management of cardiac emergencies. This includes cardioversion and defibrillation, cardiac rhythm recognition, transcutaneous pacing, airway management, intravenous (IV) treatment, and resuscitation medications. Program personnel will utilize a multidisciplinary approach that can include registered nurses, respiratory therapists, exercise specialists, occupational therapists, registered dieticians, social workers, and certified personal trainers. All members of the wellness staff are trained and regularly updated in basic life support—cardio pulmonary resuscitation (CPR). All the staff, including personal trainers, is instructed in the use of an automatic external defibrillator (AED). This devise looks at a person's heart rhythm, recognizes cardiac arrest, and talks responder through simple defibrillation steps. Continuing staff education in the health and fitness field is recommended and supported by the affiliated hospital.

The wellness program is an integral part of medical care. "In secondary prevention programs, once a patient enters the hospital with an 'event' or is given the diagnosis of diabetes or COPD, a referral is generated," says Schmidt. "We are the outpatient part of treatment. We provide the skills for medical management and lifestyle changes, as well as education about the condition. We are in regular contact with the primary medical doctor while they (clients) are in our programs." For folks with your diagnosis, the wellness program promotes independence, individual health and fitness goals, and positive results in a safe and accepting environment. "The satisfaction of watching patients change when they learn how to take care of themselves is a draw for me," says Schmidt. "They feel in control and empowered again." A wellness program is your vehicle for an optimal health outcome.

For the hospital that has a wellness program, there can be three rehabilitation phases. Phase I is for the inpatient. If you are hospitalized with a cardiac event, diabetes, or COPD, your primary care physician and any specialists working with you will initiate the education and ambulation process. If you are a diabetic client, you may receive a visit from the wellness diabetes nurse or a diabetes educator. If you are in the hospital as a result of heart disease, a cardiac nurse or exercise physiologist associated with the program will make contact with you. A respiratory therapist, pulmonary nurse, or physical therapist will touch base with you if you are a COPD patient. When a wellness staff member visits an inpatient, they will provide information about the Phase II outpatient segment of the program and may also set up an appointment at that time, but you do not have to be hospitalized to participate. You can speak with a wellness coordinator at any time about the requirements for direct admission into Phase II. If you are a candidate, your physician will be contacted for a referral and an intake appointment will be scheduled.

Phase II is the outpatient or post-diagnosis recovery and moving forward stage. This is an exciting time of learning and renewal. On a scheduled date you will meet with your wellness coordinator for an intake interview. The history of your current illness and other chronic problems, a brief physical assessment, a listing of current medications, the names of your doctors, a stress and depression assessment, and your risk factors and risk stratification will all be entered into your personal chart. You will have the opportunity to ask questions and express concerns, and you will receive detailed information about Phase II, such as length of time you will be in the program; dates, times, and subjects of scheduled education classes; and dates and times of exercise classes. Medicare allowances and other insurance coverage, which will vary according to plan, will be discussed during your intake interview.

Education is a large part of Phase II. You will be privy to a series of presentations geared to your illness. Pulmonary education may include classes on breathing techniques, types of lung problems, environmental irritants, medications, and emotions and depression. Diabetes courses can address foot care, complications, meal planning, and regulating blood glucose. Cardiac classes can be about understanding cholesterol, eating for a health heart, stress reduction, and relaxation techniques. In addition to classroom instruction, you will participate in a closely supervised fitness program with an exercise prescription designed exclusively for you and your present state of health. Once you have completed Phase II, you will have the option of participating in Phase III of wellness. This is called maintenance. It is a place for you to safely continue your exercise routine in an independent setting with the continued guidance and care of the wellness staff.

Providing tools for patients with your diagnosis, this diverse wellness program will help you sow the seeds of success. As an integral part of your medical team, it offers one-on-one meetings with staff trained in your particular diagnostic needs, educational classes geared to illness management, and disease-specific booklets and handouts. Every intake interview, classroom instruction, and meeting will be focused on your particular chronic illness, but there is one segment of the program that comprehensively embraces and

BASICS TO BRING TO INTAKE INTERVIEW

Always bring a list of your current medications including prescription, over-the-counter, and herbal therapies. Have a thorough list of questions and all insurance information with you. Bring your husband, wife, significant other, friend, or family member as an extra pair of ears. For what to bring and what questions to ask specific to your illness, see Questions and Concerns, page 118.

supports all involved clients: wellness exercise. Diagnosis, fitness level, past history notwithstanding, all cardiac, diabetes, and COPD clients are encouraged to participate in wellness exercise.

By entering a wellness fitness class, you will have the potential to improve your physical condition, create a healthy mental outlook, and maintain functional independence. In *Lifetime Fitness and Wellness*, Melvin H. Williams writes, "Often, when individuals initiate a health behavior change, experience the related benefits, and develop a personal health ethic relative to that behavior, they begin to modify other unhealthy behaviors as well. Exercise may be a key health behavior in this regard, for it may spur interest in other health behavior changes, such as a change to a healthy diet or cessation of smoking. The more healthful behavior changes you make, the greater the probability of living life to its fullest."

3

EXERCISE—THE WELLNESS PROGRAM COMMON DENOMINATOR

IN 1553, DR. CHRISTOBAL MENDEZ wrote a book devoted in its entirety to exercise. Mendez, a Spanish physician, was a proponent of walking, recommending the activity for men and women alike. He also proposed exercise for children and the handicapped. In the nineteenth century, when many Americans started moving to cities and getting away from the rugged physical demands of life on the frontier, American doctors began expressing concerns for what they saw as a growing sedentary lifestyle. People were told to exercise. Bicycling, calisthenics, walking, gymnastics, and training with dumbbells became popular activities. The "well" population wanted to stay healthy, feel more competent, and look good. On the other hand, chronic illness sufferers were advised to take their medicine and take it easy. At the time, exercise recommendations and standards for the chronically ill were nonexistent.

Dr. Kenneth H. Cooper noted changes in theories regarding exercise and chronic illness management in his best-selling book, *Aerobics*, published in 1968. Cooper writes about a Cleveland, Ohio YMCA program initiated in the late 1950's. "Cardiac cases, business men in their 50s and 60s, began running in this pioneer Y-sponsored program. And it took courage because some of them were coming off their second and third heart attacks and there was very little encouragement for this sort of thing in medical tradition. I mention this Cleveland program specifically because it was one of the few where accurate medical data were taken on the participants, before and after their exercise programs."

In his book, Cooper—who pioneered scientifically measuring the effects of vigorous activity on the body—also writes about his success with the prescription of the slowly increased exercise regime that he adapted for an Air Force pilot grounded with heart problems. He includes, too, early information on medical findings regarding exercise for lung disease. "Several doctors I know have started their lung patients into a gradual reconditioning program with encouraging success. After their condition has stabilized, the patients are strongly encouraged to get out of bed and start walking around the corridors, then up and down stairs. Some are given oxygen tanks on wheels or portable, strap-on oxygen containers and, breathing the oxygen, they walk around the hospital, and even outdoors where they perform nominal tasks around the hospital grounds." In his discussion regarding diabetes and exercise, Cooper says, "We've had most of our success with early diabetics, those not yet on shots. Many pilots with symptoms of early diabetes have been returned to flying status when a good diet, weight reduction, and a good physical-conditioning program completely controlled their diabetes." In 1970, The Cooper Institute was founded for the study and documentation of exercise and mortality relationship. It has expanded over the years to include a wide variety of research, health, fitness, and education programs.

Today, the known benefits of regular exercise are well-established. The heart works more efficiently, circulation improves, bone loss is decreased, muscle strength and endurance are increased, and there's an improvement in lipid variables that includes a reduction in bad cholesterol, low-density lipoprotein (LDL), and the increase of good cholesterol, high-density lipoprotein (HDL). With exercise, stress hormones are decreased, which can, in turn, lower blood pressure and heart rate, lessen fatigue, and improve posture and flexibility. When combined with a sound diet that reasonably limits calories, exercise promotes a healthy reduction in weight. The fit body burns fat more efficiently and shows a decrease in waist-to-hip ratio and an increase in metabolism. Exercise can enhance relaxation, reduce anxiety and stress, elevate mood, and promote a sense of well-being. Some age-related declines may also be postponed or prevented.

The exercise picture has also expanded for those people with COPD, heart disease, and diabetes. As noted in *Conn's Current Therapy*, a medical therapy text, "Rehabilitation has quickly come into vogue for the treatment of COPD. Pulmonary rehabilitation has reduced hospitalization in COPD patients. Specific guidelines for rehabilitation vary, but all stress aerobic activity." In reference to exercise for cardiac patients, the text indicates that Phase II heart patients initiate lifelong exercise and lifestyle changes. "The goals of exercise should be clear: Training will restore and increase functional capacity and effort-related symptoms will improve." The need for fitness for diabetics is also clear. *Magill's Medical Guide, Health and Illness* states, "Exercise is particularly helpful in the management of both types of diabetes, because working muscle does not require insulin to metabolize glucose. Thus, exercising muscles take up and use some of the excess glucose in the blood, which reduces the overall need for insulin." The weight loss experience that occurs as the result of regular exercise and a controlled diet will also help keep blood sugar within normal limits.

With these new findings and advances, your diagnosis makes you a prime candidate for a fitness agenda. An exercise program is vitally important for chronic diseases, says Dr. Smith-Poling. "Even ten percent more endurance can improve quality of life, and there is greater independence because they have more exercise tolerance. A supervised exercise program is one of the best ways to gain ground against chronic illness. Increasing aerobic

BENEFITS OF EXERCISE

Benefits include more efficient heart function, improved circulation, decreased bone loss, increased muscle strength and endurance, improved lipids, lowered blood pressure and heart rate, improved posture, weight loss, reduced anxiety and stress. There is reduced hospitalization for COPD patients, positive lifestyle change for cardiac patients, and controlled blood glucose and reduced overall need for insulin for the diabetic.

capacity means for any given activity you don't have to work as hard. You're in better condition. It's less work on your heart. Likewise for your lungs, you don't have to extract as much oxygen, and some patients with COPD can get by with lower oxygen because their conditioned muscles don't need as much, and if you can get a diabetic to lose weight, it will markedly improve the disease."

Wellness personal trainer Frank Gentle knows firsthand what exercise can do for chronic illness. Before he became a trainer, he had a heart attack. After undergoing major heart surgery, he participated in all three phases of the medically supervised wellness program. "When I was young, I was very active. I played every sport available, including running all the short 100 meter-200 meter events with some success," he says. "Then I got into a pattern of not regularly exercising. I was active and doing things all the time in the years before my heart attack, but as far as scheduled aerobic exercise, I didn't do that. I think you can get into a pattern of not working out until it's decided for you that you have to exercise, which was the case with me." Less than two weeks after his 1993 three-way bypass surgery, Gentle was in a Phase II cardiac exercise course. "I thought it was great," he says. "I think it was a throwback to when I was younger and exercised a whole lot more, and with wellness you're in a community of your peers, and I believe that helps." Physically, Gentle has experienced an improvement in his heart condition. "When I walk a treadmill test now the doctor stops me, whereas in the past I would have to stop. Now he says he's seen enough and everything's fine."

With your diagnosis, taking care of your own wellness by following a medically designed fitness program will regenerate your life and bolster your ability to manage the disease, and when facing a chronic illness the benefits of exercise beyond the general improvements are considerable. Exercise offers you more than physical fitness. It takes discipline to workout regularly. That self-training will carry over into daily life.

If you're dealing with diabetes, establishing a positive habit of fitness will initiate taking control of negative habits, such as smoking. The discipline will also help you develop a meal routine, get in the mode of monitoring and recording carbohydrate intake, and encourage you to pay attention to your blood sugar numbers.

If you are a heart patient, the discipline of a positive habit of fitness will initiate taking control of negative habits, such as smoking, and jump-start you into the swing of a heart-healthy diet.

If you are a pulmonary client, the discipline of a positive habit of fitness will initiate taking control of negative habits, such as smoking, and will reinforce applying new breathing techniques and proper body positions to everyday activities.

Exercise promotes feeling good. "It is clear that activity and fitness have the potential to improve mild to moderate cases of anxiety and depression," writes Sharkey in *Fitness and Health*. Exercisers with chronic illness report sleeping better, regaining a sense of control over their lives, and that they have a feeling of pride in their "new normal" accomplishments. "You definitely get a high from exercising, and emotional spirits are buoyed," adds Gentle. "As I continued on in several different programs, there was one common thread—a kindred spirit between everyone—because we all knew that we had been through something and had survived. We were all still here, and that was good." Becoming a wellness personal trainer is a natural transition for Gentle. It helps him to continue with exercise, talk to people about it, and bestow his expertise. "Sometimes you wonder what you have in this world. What do you bring to the table? The one thing I have is that I can talk to people and show them what I know," he says. "What I know as far as exercise is very positive, and I talk from personal experience. My life after the heart attack and surgery has been on an upward curve. I share my experience. A wellness exercise program can extend not just life, but living."

Exercising for health requires a lifetime commitment, but the road must be navigated one day at a time. "Working with chronic disease is frustrating for the doctor as well as the patient," says Smith-Poling. "Everyone wants a long-term cure, but sometimes you just have to take today. You can either have a terrible attitude about life, or you can enjoy every flower."

4

WELLNESS EXERCISE— A DIFFERENT BALLGAME

Do You Fit with Fitness?

EXERCISE. THE VERY THOUGHT sends you running for the nearest recliner. There, under the cozy folds of a favorite afghan, you read, knit, do crosswords, push the television remote buttons and wait for the outlandish "fitness for health" concept to pass. For you, exercise is something to get out of doing. And you are a member of a creative group. When physical education was mandatory in high school, you and your cohorts had a steady stream of the best and most plausible pardons. From dramatic gyrations miming pounding migraines and the mother lode of abdominal cramps, to being the only audiovisual aide students able to fix a defunct projector, you artistically avoided all but the required gym classes. As an adult perpetuating your adversity to physical training, as far as you're concerned, Nike is a Greek goddess, sweat pants make good dust rags and car wipes, gyms are for jocks (and jocks are deranged), and your dialogue is compelling. "My mother was ninety-nine when she died. She ate eggs every morning, drank beer every night, and never exercised a day in her life." In light of your illness, you are willing to adjust to downing pills, rearranging your diet, poking holes in your fingers, or puffing inhalers, but you remain a staunch exercise nonbeliever. Eluding a workout at every turn, you take your diagnosis to the couch.

On the flip side, you may be a former athlete: a linebacker, marathon runner, track star, mountain climber, weight lifter, or tennis pro in your day. If so, you are a devotee to fitness to the extreme, a member of the "no pain no gain" fragment of society.

A retired personal trainer or two may join you in this category, remembering what it was like to be at the top of their game and tackling the onset of illness by getting whipped back into shape with an accelerated (and sometimes dangerous) exercise drill. Re-incarnating the devil-may-care demeanor of indestructible youth, with your new diagnosis you hit the dirt running. First it's a few laps around the track, just like the old days. If you survive the run, it's on to some hardcore weightlifting and fifty sit ups followed by a crawl to the nearest bed, the warmest heating pad, and often the end of all exercise until your body and mind recoup.

Possibly, you fall into yet a third category. You may be the busy bee. Lively and animated with an active style, you walk the dog, tend the garden, golf, push a vacuum, stack the wood pile, and play in the park with grandchildren. Substituting tasks and hobbies for a scheduled workout, you fill the day with motion and say you get plenty of exercise. Touting personal satisfaction, a sense of accomplishment, and maintained flexibility as benefits of being industrious, with a daily list of completed chores under your belt you exempt yourself from a planned, prolonged workout on the assumption that a mobile life precludes the need for a formal fitness program.

In truth, all three fitness scenarios have a plus side. Good genes can carry the non-exerciser a long way. The fitness zealot has a lot going for them in enthusiasm and inclination. The active person benefits from the regular dose of physical movement and completed jobs. Even under the best circumstances, however, these behaviors have little to offer when it comes to long-term muscular strength and endurance. Add a diagnosis of heart disease, diabetes, or COPD to the picture and all three exercise viewpoints can be detrimental.

Everyone has the potential for physical improvement with on-going training, but with a chronic illness you stand to reap enormous, life-enhancing benefits by pursuing fitness through a wellness exercise class. Dissecting your exercise attitudes and replacing misconceptions with facts is a good way to get started.

EXERCISER AVOIDER

You have come to terms with your diagnosis. You're making dietary changes, have lost a little weight, and are adjusting to the barrage of new procedures and medications—but you are not exercising. By now, the incessant prodding from your doctors, family members, and friends to get involved in an organized workout arrangement is grating on your nerves. As you've come to understand your illness, the short and long-term advantages of a regular fitness regime may be tweaking you intellectually, but physically and emotionally you hang onto the notion that joining a class is not for you. "I knew I had to exercise to get better, but at first I wanted to go it alone," admits one reformed avoider. "The thought of being in a gym with all those complicated machines and barely covered hard bodies was intimidating. I was sure I'd look dumb and stand out like a sore thumb. As it turned out, I never did do it on my own." In the interest of improved health, let's keep that workout room door ajar. As an exercise avoider, you are a good candidate for a regularly scheduled course, and there could be reasons beyond a stronger body and better management of your illness that will convince you to give the idea of wellness fitness a chance.

WHAT'S IN IT FOR YOU?

There are no Schwarzenegger wannabes. You will work at a comfortable pace suited to your needs and capabilities. Assistance will be readily available. There will be diversion from exercise through conversation and companionship. You will have a schedule. You will be in an atmosphere conducive to continuation and improvement.

First, let's dispel some myths. Cardiac, diabetes, COPD wellness facilities are not generic gyms. No one is scantly clad in thong bikinis, not even the instructors. The dress code is comfortable, loose clothing and supportive shoes. The others in the class will be in the same boat as you. There are no Schwarzenegger wannabes bulking up in front of the mirrors, and the only competition will be in telling the funniest joke or having the best photos of grandkids. You will be exercising within the parameters of a plan designed to be specific to your needs and capabilities, and you will be encouraged to progress at a pace that works comfortably for you. You will not be left to sink or swim on your own. A staff member will always be available to assist you with the machines, you will be regularly monitored, and if you have health concerns or questions, a nurse or appropriately trained staff person will work with you.

Putting aside the fact that you will have to exercise consistently in order to experience lower blood sugars, a stronger heart muscle, or better functioning lungs, the structure of a wellness group will be a strong factor for your continued motivation. Being a person prone to eluding exercise, a class is the best place for you. Most non-athletic types who bite the bullet and decide to go the solo route to fitness discontinue within the first six months. One reason may be that when exercising alone, the disdain for the activity is paramount, and the negative internal dialogue becomes louder and stronger than a shaky decision to get fit. As a member of a class, a couch potato often finds that the conversation and companionship become the larger part of the focus. New friendships are formed, information is shared, and there are like minds in the "What, you expect me to exercise?" mindset to commiserate with. One avid avoider says, "It's a fast hour of the dreaded 'E' word. Even though I know it's good for me, I would stop after five minutes without people to talk to." Also, there is commitment to schedule. If the class is noted on the calendar every Monday, Wednesday, and Friday, there's a tendency to show up, if not for the workout, for the social and psychological benefits. But in the flurry of distractions, don't lose sight of a subsequent gain. Be sure to keep an eye on the state of your physical health. Your improvements may change your attitude about the "E" word.

FORMER ATHLETE

If you are a positive-fitness former athlete with heart disease, diabetes, or COPD, you may be saving your life by joining wellness exercise, or, at the very least, preventing injury. For you a workout once meant pushing to the max, challenging the mind and body, mastering the next course. In your day, the stimulation of bettering your personal best far outweighed the pain of screaming muscles. As a marathoner, you ran through the discomfort of an aching back, throbbing knees, blistering feet, and blackened toenails. Hitting the wall meant reaching the stupor of exhaustion then pushing beyond—calling up the courage to transcend. If you were the tennis buff, you played with sore elbows and taped knees and lobed through head colds and allergies. But this is a different ballgame.

There's trouble brewing if you maintain an attitude of more-is-better when combining exercise and chronic illness. If you try to master the problem without looking at the illness-related ramifications,

---

WHAT'S IN IT FOR YOU?

You will prevent injury and learn illness-related ramifications of excessive exercise. New habits will be established to get the most out of exercise. There will be the availability of good tools and trained experts. You will have the potential to master your illness.

---

you will find yourself in a pattern of taking ten steps forward and five back. If you're dealing with diabetes, it is imperative to know your body's glucose variations in connection with different levels of activity. You will want to measure blood glucose before and after exercise, learn the symptoms of low and high sugar and how to recognize them during a workout, and establish eating habits that mesh with your body and its response to exercise. If you are a cardiac patient taking heart-related medications called beta blockers, your heart's response to exercise will be altered, making the monitoring of heart rate an inaccurate measure of workout intensity. You will have to learn a new method of determining how hard you're working. It will also be important to become familiar with your body's signals in relation to angina pain. If COPD is your issue, to get the most out of exercise you will want to establish new breathing techniques, find the best time of day for your aerobic activity, be aware of how much oxygen is saturating your hemoglobin, and learn to judge how hard you're breathing in a variety of activity levels.

In the area of fitness, the most efficient way to gain control over your illness is to acknowledge its existence, learn how your new body conditions respond to a controlled and monitored workout, and then use all available tools to get the most out of exercise while avoiding the pitfalls of old habits. The wellness exercise program has the tools and trained experts to guide you toward a rewarding, challenging, and safe "new normal" fitness life. To be successful, self-sufficient, and safe, the best you can be is a heartbeat away. With the take-charge mentality of a positive-fitness person, you will have the potential to master your illness.

BUSY BEE

Can there be opportunities for the busy bee in a wellness class? With your bustling schedule, you may not think so, but think again. Your daily activities are wonderful and should be continued, but are they giving you an adequate workout? Doctors recommend at least twenty to thirty minutes of sustained aerobic exercise a day (at least three times a week) to achieve fitness benefits. What that boils down to is that while the latest findings suggest it is no longer necessary to do an entire thirty minutes all at once to get aerobic benefit (you can do fifteen minutes in the morning and another fifteen in the afternoon), it is necessary to maintain an aerobic pace during each division. Walking the dog doesn't do much for your body aerobically. It's a great outing for both of you, a wonderful boost to morale, and adds a lot to keeping you agile, but walking a few steps between stops at every bush doesn't cut it for aerobic fitness. This is the case with most household chores, hobbies, and outdoor ventures. Vacuuming and yard work employ stop-and-go movements. If you walk nine or all eighteen holes on the golf course, you are adding to mobility and flexibility, but you're not likely at any point to segue into a brisk fifteen minute stride. With this information, if you're thinking that you'll just add a sustained speed walk to your current schedule, it is important to note that not everyone with a diagnosis of diabetes, COPD, or heart disease is a candidate for that amount of aerobic activity, at least not initially. You will need to scrutinize your body's response to prolonged exercise.

In joining wellness, you will see your capacity, learn your limits, and get to know your physical state in relation to your illness. At first, you may have to put a chore or two aside to accommodate your new workout and to give yourself a chance to adjust. As you grow stronger and have a better handle on your illness, you may be able to put your sidelined enterprises back in the schedule, or combine one of them with your workout. For example, get Rover involved in fitness. A busy bee diabetes wellness client learned how to include a speed walk in her daily scheme. Shortening her leisurely stroll with the dog, she added a twenty minute non-stop trek that she could do with her pet. "It works out great now that I know what they mean by aerobic exercise," she says. "On one of the days that I don't go to class, I take my dog, Max, to a grassy area first so he's relieved, and then we go to the beach for our faster pace. Max is really into it, too, and we've both lost weight. Once I got use to it, I found I had a lot more energy."

WHAT'S IN IT FOR YOU?

You will learn the difference between chores and an aerobic workout. You will learn how to set aside time for true aerobic exercise. You will see how your body responds to prolonged exercise and to a more strenuous workout in a safe environment. You will see your capacity, learn limits, and get to know your physical state in relation to your illness. You will learn ways to incorporate an aerobic routine into your daily schedule.

Under the direction of the trained wellness staff, you will be guided through a progressive fitness program that will accommodate your state of health, account for activity limitations, and complement your current pleasures. This approach will afford you the opportunity to adapt to a more strenuous workout and improve functional independence in a safe environment. You will learn ways to incorporate fitness into your busy schedule and develop better health for the continued enjoyment of all daily events.

What makes avoiders, former athletes, and busy bees successful members of a wellness exercise class? You all share a similar boot-in-the-pants experience, and no matter your view of physical activity, you will step up to the plate and catch life's curve ball. Like all wellness participants, you are fighters, believers, seekers, and teachers. You turn wrestle into wisdom, angst into assurance, and a diagnosis into direction.

—>●<—

5

BASIC WELLNESS EXERCISE

EQUIPMENT, ACTIVITIES, TECHNIQUES, SAFETY

EVERYDAY LIFE PASSES unnoticed until an intrusion colors the norm with gray confusion. A chronic health problem disrupts the ordinary with perplexing physical and mental change. It picks you up and puts you down in strange environs. Even the positive adjustments you initiate in the management of your illness can be daunting. A wellness fitness program is new territory. Exploring the terrain will replace muddle with muscle. To move forward with a feeling of control, let's look at the basics of wellness exercise before your first workout. Keep in mind that when you do start, you will be working with a staff member on an exercise plan designed around your current needs and future potential.

The three basic types of exercise that you will be doing are aerobic (cardiovascular), range of motion (flexibility), and resistance (muscle strengthening). Aerobic exercise can be vigorous, but shouldn't be done to the point of being out of breath. If there's not enough oxygen to meet the physical demands, the exercise becomes anaerobic. Walking and bicycling are aerobic activities. You will work on improving flexibility and range of motion by employing a variety of stretches. For resistance, you will do isotonic exercises. Isotonic means exercising against a movable resistance. This can include weight training and the use of resistance bands. Isometric resistive exercises (working against an immovable object) can cause a rise in blood pressure and are generally not used in this wellness setting.

The amount and variation of equipment in your location will

depend on program budget, available space, and number of participants. There will be machines that provide an aerobic or cardiovascular workout. In that regard, most wellness gyms will have treadmills. A treadmill is a motorized, weight-bearing machine used for indoor walking. Holding onto a handrail for support, you walk on a rubber tread that rotates from front to back. The speed is controlled by pushing a button or arrow up or down. There will also be a control button or arrow to create an incline, as well as one for an emergency stop.

Stationary upright bicycles are gym staples for aerobic activity. The Schwinn Airdyne is a popular model. The handlebars move in conjunction with the pedals, so you reap both upper and lower body benefits. The Airdyne has a fan in the front wheel that creates self-generating air resistance. Stationary upright bike models without movable handlebars are also used in wellness gyms. As with regular street bicycles, the upright bike pedals are under your feet with circular, up-and-down leg movement. Upright bicycle seats adjust to different

TYPES OF WELLNESS EXERCISE

Aerobic (cardiovascular), range of motion (flexibility), and resistance (muscle strengthening). Resistance is an isotonic exercise. This means working against a movable resistance.

heights. Another bike style is the recumbent. It has the benefit of a wide, padded seat and tilted, padded back support. The seat adjusts forward and back to suit leg length, and the machine is lower to the to the floor than the upright bike, making getting on and off fairly easy. When you sit on a recumbent bike, the pedals are in front of you and have a circular, forward-and-back motion. There are stationary handgrips on either side of the seat. Most facilities will have one NUSTEP recumbent bicycle (some will have more). This style has the added benefit of adjustable handlebars that move with the pedals. Like the other recumbent bikes, it has a tilted back support, and the wide, padded seat moves forward and back to accommodate leg length. The NUSTEP seat also unlocks to rotate left or right for easy on and off maneuvering. Arm rests that lift add to the user-friendly style. With the addition of the handlebar movement on the NUSTEP, you can achieve a satisfying upper and lower body workout. Recumbent bikes give good support to the body and are ideal for people who are not ready or able to use other machines. There is adjustable tension on the recumbent bicycles.

Cross trainers or elliptical trainers simulate walking without the body-pounding component of actually taking steps. The standing position is weight bearing, but there is no impact to the body. There are two steps for your feet and two hand bars. You employ a striding motion and the steps and hand bars move with your gait (some models may not have movable hand bars). Elliptical trainers have resistance adjustments to increase or decrease the tension. Step machines replicate stair climbing, also minus the pounding. On some machines the hand grips are stationary and on others the grips move with the steps. The up and down pedaling is generated by pushing one leg down after the other. Step machines have resistance adjustments.

Rowers do just what the name implies, and if the wellness facility has a water view the imagination can catapult you back to youthful summers on the lake. The rower is quite low to the floor and the seat moves easily (you can place a chair to the side of the machine for support while getting on and off). Stepping over the center bar, you lower yourself onto the seat and place feet in the two supports in front of you. On most models, there will be straps to secure your feet. Picking up the center hand bar that will be attached to a chain pulley, you simulate a rowing motion by pushing against the foot supports and sliding back on the seat until your legs are almost straight out in front of you. At the same time you're pulling the bar toward your chest. Sliding forward, bending the knees and extending arms (and hand bar), the motion is reversed. The rower has a resistance adjustment.

Your wellness gym may have a hand cycle. This machine works the upper body and can be set up on a table or a low, wide, sturdy wall shelf. The hand cycle is easy to use, and is ideal if you suffer from claudication (pain or cramping) in your legs or buttocks that occurs with exertion, or have neuropathy (deterioration of nerve fiber, especially in diabetic feet). Sitting on a chair (or in a wheelchair) facing the machine, you use arms and shoulders to rotate two handgrips. Movement is at your own speed, and the arm resistance is adjusted to your comfort.

Most of the aerobic equipment in a wellness gym will have computer displays with information such as speed, distance, time, workload level, revolutions per minute (RPM), metabolic equivalents (METS), calories burned, heart rate, and power output (WATTS). The machines may also have computerized program options for variations in workout intensity, but the wellness personnel usually stick to their own system of manually entering personalized exercise prescriptions specific to the medical and physical needs of each individual.

AEROBIC EXERCISE EQUIPMENT

In a wellness gym, treadmills, stationary and recumbent bicycles, rowers, stair steppers, elliptical machines, and hand cycles provide a cardiovascular (aerobic) workout.

Many facilities include the use of resistance bands or tubing, exercise balls, and abdominal crunch machines in their workout plan. The bands (isotonic training) have handles at each end and come in several different color-coded resistance levels. There are standing and sitting resistance band actions that are used to increase muscle strength and endurance and improve range of motion and flexibility. The exercise balls are good for stretching, balance, and coordination. Positions for ball use vary according to desired outcome and ability to safely carry out maneuvers. The abdominal crunch machine (isotonic training) helps tighten and strengthen abdominal muscles. Sitting with your back against a padded rest, you grasp the overhead handles and pull them forward, using your abdominal muscles to curl the upper body around the stomach and slowly roll back to an upright position. You repeat the curling and rolling-back movement for a prescribed number of repetitions. Weights on the back or side of the crunch machine are lifted in conjunction with the movement. You control the amount of weight lifted. In most cases, this is accomplished by inserting a metal pin between a stack of attached weights that are marked for size. Sometimes, the weights are manually placed on a long bar connected to the side or on the back of the device. If you have not used the abdominal crunch, but are interested in trying it out, you should confer with the staff. It is not for everybody, especially people with certain types of back, neck, and shoulder problems. If you do use it, you will be instructed in correct form and appropriate weight.

At first, a lot of the gym paraphernalia may not be part of your general procedure, and it may be that some of it will never be recommended. The equipment that is prescribed will be compatible with your workout proficiency given your current state of health. With continued exercise and improved conditioning, new machines and an increase in workout intensity may well be added to your menu. For some newly diagnosed people, the first days of wellness aerobic exercise may be a slow, easy walk around the gym.

You will be encouraged to stretch (range of motion/flexibility). This is not the same as warming up. A warm-up readies the body for more rigorous activity and reduces risk of injury. A warm-up is accomplished by starting with a slow first five minutes at whatever aerobic activity begins your session. Stretching is done after your aerobic work when muscles are warm and pliable and there is an increase in blood flow. Stretching increases range of motion and flexibility, decreases soreness, and helps to get oxygen and other nutrients to muscle tissue. It is best to practice static, or passive, stretching. This entails moving slowly into position until you feel an easy, relaxed pull in the focused muscle. If you feel pain, you'll be advised to easy up on the stretch. With static stretching, the position is held for ten to fifteen seconds without bouncing.

BANDS, ABDOMINAL MACHINES, & BALLS

Resistance bands and abdominal machines are isotonic (exercising against a movable resitance) forms of training used for strengthening muscles. Exercise balls improve flexibility, balance, and coordination.

Bouncing, which is called ballistic stretching, causes muscles to contract rather than expand.

You will learn a basic routine for stretching your upper and lower body. Upper body movements will involve your arm, shoulder, chest, back, and neck muscles. Hands and fingers can also be worked. You may do easy side bends that work the oblique muscles and a knee-to-chest movement that helps the lower back. There will be a variety of leg stretches for hamstrings, quadriceps, calves, ankles, feet, and toes. To accommodate your present recovery status, the stretches will be executed in both standing and seated positions. Occasionally, floor mats and exercise balls may be used for stretching.

STRETCHING

Stretching is done after an aerobic workout. It increases range of motion and flexibility, decreases soreness, and gets oxygen to muscle tissue. Static stretching that involves holding each position for ten-to-fifteen seconds without bouncing is advised. You will learn both upper and lower body stretches.

Your workout will include weight training with hand-held weights. Weight training is isotonic (exercising against a movable resistance). It firms and strengthens muscles and increases endurance. Everybody should weight train, but don't panic. Wellness weight training won't produce bulging biceps and enormous pecs, and you won't be greasing up for national weightlifting competitions. What you will be doing is building and maintaining physical independence by increasing muscle endurance and coordination. Remaining independent means having the ability to handle such everyday tasks and pleasures as working in the yard, hoisting groceries out of the car and reaching to put them away, maneuvering in and out of the bathtub, and lifting a cherished grandchild. For this type of training, light hand weights will be used, with a focus on increasing the number of repetitions.

When you are starting out with weights, the staff will want you to be conservative, perhaps using just one or two pounds for four to six repetitions. This enables the nurses and trainers to assess your form and breathing, as well as note any discomfort you may experience during each lift. You are training for endurance. This means using reasonably light weights while focusing, over time, on adding more repetitions to your workout. Depending on your risk factors, your trainer may initiate a gradual increase to twelve repetitions. Any increase in the size of the hand weights you use will also be gradual and not excessive.

Weight training can be carried out in a standing or sitting position. If standing, you will be advised on proper posture, which will include keeping your knees slightly bent and pelvis tilted forward to take pressure off your back, maintaining a loose grip on the weights, and watching that your body doesn't sway when the weight is lifted. Whether standing or sitting, if your arm muscles twitch or shake while doing any type of extensions away from your body, the wellness trainer will suggest a lighter weight, or recommend doing that particular motion with no weight at all until your strength increases. Don't rush through the weightlifting. Raising the weights to a count of two and lowering to a count of four is a good formula to follow. As you get stronger and can do twelve repetitions of each lift in your routine, your trainer may encourage you to increase the amount of weight you use. With

WEIGHT TRAINING

Weight training is isotonic (exercising against a movable resistance). If standing, keep knees slightly bent and pelvis tilted forward. Avoid body swaying. Maintain a loose grip, and reduce size of weights if muscles tremble or twitch during lifts. Lift and lower weights slowly, and remember to breathe. Four to six repetitions is a good start. Twelve comfortable repetitions of each lift for several weeks is a good goal before increasing amount of weight. Increase by one pound only and decrease lifts by half for the first week or two with the heavier weight. Three times a week (not on consecutive days) is a good weight training schedule. Stop if you have pain.

hand weights, any increase will be initiated in one-pound incre-
ments. When this occurs, the number of your repetitions will be
cut in half for the first week or two, then you may gradually add
repetitions again. If you feel any discomfort, stop the activity and
consult with the wellness staff.

How you breathe during weight training is important. People
have a tendency to hold their breath when they lift weights. Doing this elevates blood pressure. The ideal breathing technique is
to exhale on the lift or the exertive movement and inhale on the
downward motion. At first this will seem odd and difficult to do,
but it can become habit with practice. If you find yourself spend-
ing a lot of time trying to master this breathing style, it is okay to
just breathe regularly. As the staff will reinforce, the idea is to avoid
holding your breath. Weight training three times a week (not on
consecutive days) is recommended, but you will be advised on the
best application of your program. A total-body weight training
workout can be accomplished with hand weights.

During the Phase II exercise segment of wellness, cardiac clients,
and in some programs COPD clients, are monitored through the
use of a telemetry system. Telemetry is the transmission of the
heart's rhythm to a receiving station for analysis. Connection is
simple and noninvasive. Two adhesive-backed disks with components for snap-in clips are applied; one goes on the upper right
side of the chest near your shoulder and the other on the lower
left side of your torso. Electrodes, attached to a small transmitter, are snapped into the disks. The transmitter is hooked to your
clothing, or you can place it in a shirt pocket. Through the telemetry system, the staff monitors your heart rhythm before, during,
and after exercise from the telemetry computer screen display.
Telemetry is not used in Phase III maintenance.

A pulse oximeter is used in both Phase II and in many of the
maintenance classes. Primarily for COPD clients, pulse oximetry
is a noninvasive means of detecting the percentage of hemoglobin
that is saturated with oxygen. A probe attached to a small computerized unit is placed on a fingertip or ear lobe. The computer displays
the percent of oxygen saturation and pulse rate. Ideally, your oxygen saturation number should be above ninety during exercise. For

those pulmonary exercisers who maintain good saturations during a workout, the pulse oximeter helps them to see that they are in a safe range and can try increasing intensity a bit more.

The typical wellness facility will have charts displayed in various locations around the gym. They can include stretching guides and a formula for easy heart rate determination. The rate of perceived exertion (RPE) and rate of perceived dyspnea (RPD) charts (see inside covers) that help assign a value to the intensity of a workout will be posted near the machines. Often, the nurses and trainers have smaller versions of these charts with them as they move through the gym to check on each exerciser. The rate of perceived exertion chart has numbers on one side and descriptions of physical exertion levels on the other. During your time on each machine, the class facilitator will ask about the intensity of your workout. You will evaluate how you physically feel (legs heavy, muscles a little tired, getting hard to talk) and based on the chart, choose a number that represents how hard you feel you are working (in this case, fourteen—somewhat hard). If you have COPD, the same technique is applied to your breathing. The rate of perceived dyspnea chart has numbers on one side and breathing exertion levels on the other. When asked, you will define your breathing with a number, such as eleven—fairly easy to breathe.

TELEMETRY

Telemetry, the transmission of heart rhythm to a receiving station, will be used to monitor cardiac patients during exercise.

PULSE OXIMETER

The pulse oximeter detects the percentage of hemoglobin saturated with oxygen and will be used to determine oxygen status of clients with lung problems.

A discussion about basic wellness exercise would not be complete without addressing stress. "Although for many people stress is the spice of life, it can also be the kiss of death. Just as stress can undermine psychological contentment, it can also erode physical health and well-being. Indeed, many medical researchers believe that stress may be the greatest single contributor to disease," writes Dianne Hales in *An Invitation to Health*. Practicing simple relaxation techniques helps to manage stress. Relaxation and stress-reduction are part of wellness exercise. Some programs will have a relaxation session one day a week, possibly in place of weight training. Other facilities may incorporate it into each day of exercise, ending all classes with a few moments of gentle breathing, for example. Whatever the system, relaxation is an important component of your new routine. Whether it is quiet meditation, a guided visualization that focuses the mind on something calming, breathing exercises, or a progressive relaxation that decreases muscle tension, the staff will keep it simple, easy, and worthwhile. Once you have graduated out of Phase II and are a member of an ongoing wellness maintenance class, you may find that the group relaxation becomes a cooperative, creative venture. "Sometimes we just decide to talk and laugh," says one long-standing attendee. "We even get our nurse and trainer laughing and relaxing." Dick, a Phase II cardiac graduate and maintenance exerciser, prefers having a story or article read for relaxation. "For me, meditations are like listening to a sermon in church—I'm asleep immediately—but a short story or uplifting magazine article leaves me with a pleasant feeling. I go away with a smile on my face."

As a participant of wellness exercise, you will have the opportunity to work toward optimal fitness and health in a protected environment with qualified personnel providing assistance and information. In keeping with the secure atmosphere, *you* can safeguard the program as well. By following some basic guidelines, each exerciser can contribute to the welfare not only of themselves, but of everyone else. Safety is an integral part of the wellness experience.

When you begin your program, the staff will demonstrate proper operation of all the machines that you will be working on. As new equipment is introduced, correct use will be shown. Follow the instructions carefully, even as you become more comfortable and accustomed to the drill. If you forget how to use any piece of equipment, ask for help. For added safety, wear supportive shoes with backs and shoelace or Velcro closures. If you want to remove a sweater or shirt during your aerobic workout, stop the machine first.

In between using hand weights, avoid placing them on chairs, tables, or countertops. It is very easy for a weight to roll off the furniture and onto toes. Also, do not leave hand weights in any high traffic floor area where someone can trip over them. The gym will have a specific place to store the weights appropriately when not in use.

When doing stretches seated on an exercise ball, you can add support and prevent falls by placing a chair on either side of the ball. If you accidentally roll right or left, you can stop yourself from falling by placing a hand on the chair seat. Exercise balls should not be thrown and are to be stored away from high traffic areas when not in use. When you are working with resistance bands, allow ample room between you and others using the bands. Also, hold the handles securely. If you use a mat to do floor stretches, put the mat away after each use.

Diabetes clients who check blood glucose before and after exercise should use the designated testing area. Always dispose of lancets in a regulation receptacle. To prevent contamination, apply a small bandage to the test area. Anyone using oxygen should make cannula adjustments and liter settings before starting on a machine. If it is necessary to make changes during the workout,

SAFETY

Follow instructions regarding operation of equipment, and ask for help when necessary. Wear supportive shoes. When removing sweaters during workout, stop the machine. Make cannula adjustments and liter settings before starting exercise. Use the designated area for blood glucose testing, dispose of lancets properly, and apply a bandage to the test area. Stow belongings away from the central gym area. Do not wear perfume or aftershave. Do not use equipment without staff present.

stop the machine or ask a staff member to assist you.

Stow coats, bags, and parcels out of the central gym area. Place walkers and canes out of the way when not in use, and always watch your step when moving about the gym. To prevent skids and falls near drinking fountains, water coolers, and in bathrooms, keep water off the floor. To avoid spills in the gym area, don't leave cups of water on machines, chairs, or tabletops. Do not wear perfume or aftershave to class. The odor can cause serious breathing complications for pulmonary clients, as well as allergic reactions in those people who are susceptible. Exercise clients should not use wellness gym equipment without a staff member present.

In accordance with individual state health regulations, many wellness gyms are required to use germicidal disposable wipes to clean equipment after each use. An efficient way to do this is to have clients be responsible for a quick swab of each machine and each set of weights as they finish using them. If this is the rule of thumb in your facility, there will be disposable wipes in various locations around the gym. Latex-free, disposable gloves can also be made available to folks with allergies to cleansers and latex.

If you recognize any additional safety issues, alert the staff. If you have questions, ask. If you develop any unusual symptoms, such as dizziness, shortness of breath, chest pain, lightheadedness, or nausea, be forthcoming with the staff. These are not symptoms to ignore, and the idea of trying to exercise through them is dangerous. Tell the nurse, therapist, or trainer immediately. The issue may be one that is easily solved by slowing down, increasing oxygen, rehydrating, or resting for a few minutes— or it may be an early warning of something more serious. For your safety and well-being, let the staff determine how to handle the situation.

Your wellness center may be large and bursting at the seams with state-of-the-art machines, or it may be a small, no-frills facility with only the necessary equipment. Whatever the setting, the most important part of the gym will be you. And you are ready.

6

EXERCISING FOR LIFE WITH HEART DISEASE

CARDIAC WELLNESS EXERCISE PHASE II

"A journey of a thousand miles begins with a single step."

AS YOUR HEART HEALS and your body strengthens, you begin to venture beyond the confines of illness, and the trek is different than any past undertaking. The new terrain involves jockeying medications and side effects, conforming to a heart-healthy diet, and handling undertones of niggling confusion. Appreciation for life mixes with the apprehension of vulnerability. Aches and pains have new meaning. Is it angina or just a sore muscle; another bout of indigestion or another heart attack? If you ignore it, will it go away? New emotions buffet your spirit, and uncertainty is paramount. "Since my heart attack, I can break down and cry over a dead raccoon in the road or a sappy movie," says a burly forty-nine-year-old roofer. "It's embarrassing. I never know what will set me off. I don't want to think about any of it." Even if you choose to "bypass" the facts and try to return to life as usual, the reality will be just under the surface. Something has happened to your heart.

Registered nurse Amber Benner notes that while some of her patients express concern for a repeat heart attack and even death when starting an exercise program, many folks take heart problems too lightly. "Technology has made heart disease easily 'fixed.' Gone are the days of week-long hospitalizations and multiple restrictions on activity," Benner says. "Don't get me wrong, an overnight stay for an angioplasty/stent is much easier on the patient, but it is also easier to get back into the routine—the same routine that proliferated the heart disease. There has to be recognition that heart disease is serious and can kill you. Patients must address their risk factors and slow the progression of the disease."

Benner transitioned from intensive care nurse to wellness cardiac rehabilitation coordinator. "After many years as an ICU nurse, helping patients avoid hospitalization was a natural step. Teaching patients about their heart disease and supporting them to modify their risk factors is more satisfying than doing damage control after the heart attack," she says.

Whether you regard your illness as serious and unsettling or no big deal, being diagnosed with heart disease is the beginning of an unplanned excursion, and it can be one of your greatest adventures. Give room to your feelings, acknowledge them—good and bad—and then choose new direction over denial and fear. Take your single step and begin a worthwhile journey toward expanded knowledge and improved health. Cardiac wellness exercise is a good place to start. Close monitoring and a well-trained staff will analyze symptoms and discern problems from non-problems, there will be fellow travelers to commiserate with, and getting involved in regularly scheduled classes will provide the structure to assure that exercise happens. On the other side of that structure, the variety of equipment, the altering of speeds and times on machines to address the body's reaction to activity, segments of relaxation and stress reduction, and a focus on living instead of winning will give the competitive, impatient, perfectionist type A personality (often prone to heart attack) the opportunity to incorporate flexibility and patience into their life.

Your first cardiac exercise session will likely be conducted in a one-on-one setting before entering an established class. Exercise target heart rate will be determined to ensure that you are working aerobically. The standard target heart rate formula of 220 minus age to find maximum rate with that number multiplied by fifty-five up to eight-five percent is used. If your resting heart rate is normally fast or slow, or if you are taking a medication that regulates heart rate, such as a beta blocker, that formula will not work well. If that's the case, your blood pressure will be taken and correlated with rate of perceived exertion. "If they've had a formal treadmill test, an individualized target heart rate can be calculated with that," says Benner. Frequency, intensity, and amount of time will also be determined as part of your exercise prescription. Workout frequency for cardiac clients is three to five times a week. Suggested exercise time is thirty to sixty minutes, and it can be cumulative. Exercise intensity should be fairly light to somewhat hard in accordance with the rate of perceived exertion (RPE) chart (see inside covers). The chart, which helps to assign a value to a workout, has numbers on one side and descriptions of physical exertion levels on the other. During your time on each machine, the class facilitator will ask about the intensity of your workout. You will evaluate how you feel physically (legs heavy, muscles a little tired, getting hard to talk) and follow the chart to give a number: fourteen—somewhat hard.

At your one-on-one exercise appointment, as well as in a regular class, you will be monitored by telemetry. This enables the staff to watch your heart. Two small adhesive-backed disks that have a component for a snap-in clip are applied to the torso. One is placed on the upper right side of the chest near the shoulder, the other on the lower left side. Electrodes attached to a small transmitter are snapped into the disks. The transmitter can be hooked on a shirt or slid into a pocket. Your heart activity before, during, and after exercise will appear on the telemetry computer screen.

Before beginning your aerobic work, a wellness staff member will take a resting blood pressure. During each session, your workout activity and vitals will be recorded. Measurements can include heart rate, blood pressure, equipment used and amount of time, warm-up and working speed, power output (WATTS), metabolic equivalents (METS), size of dumbbells used for weightlifting, and all rates of perceived exertion (RPE). Medically pertinent information, as well as staff notes, will also be documented.

LET'S SPEND A WEEK in cardiac wellness exercise. There will be similarities and differences from program to program, but by coming along on this excursion you'll get a jump-start on the basics. This particular course comprises one-hour sessions held three times a week.

It's Monday, and cardiac rehab classes are underway coast to coast. On this particular morning, one new person is joining an ongoing class. The atmosphere is upbeat and pleasant. The nurse introduces the newcomer, and his classmates welcome him to the group. With brisk conversation, the established exercisers begin adeptly applying their own telemetry disks and electrodes. Dick, a Phase II graduate and wellness maintenance participant, remembers his first day of class. "It was about what you would expect in any new situation—observe, learn, adjust, and fit in. I enjoyed it and continue to look forward to regularly participating in my current exercise class." The nurse reviews the procedure of applying the telemetry disks and electrodes with the new gentleman. A wellness personal trainer starts taking resting blood pressures. The nurse checks each person in individually on the telemetry computer, records blood pressures, and asks each participant how they are and if there are any new health issues or concerns to report. Folks head for the machines.

The trainer circulates to be sure everyone is remembering to do their five-minute warm-up while the nurse works with the newest class member. Getting him started on the NUSTEP, the recumbent bike that provides both an upper and lower body workout, she explains the rate of perceived exertion (RPE) chart and how he can use it to evaluate his workout.

"It's too quiet in here," says a gentleman on one of the treadmills. "How about some lively music?"

The trainer puts on a CD of forties and fifties hits.

"Now those tunes are oldies and goodies," a woman on an Airdyne bicycle chimes in. The staff starts taking exercise blood pressures and asks how hard people feel they are working. Referring to the RPE chart posted on the wall, responses run from eleven—fairly light—to fourteen—somewhat hard.

Conversation is light and entertaining—jokes, funny happenings, pet antics, the latest diet craze—but there is underlying dialog from the nurse and trainer that focuses on client welfare. They address each exerciser with specific questions. They want to know if the gentleman on the treadmill is experiencing any angina pain with the slight increase in his walking speed. The woman on the Airdyne bike is queried about leg pain. The nurse asks the woman pedaling a recumbent bike if she's having any difficulties with her new medication. All the while, close attention is paid to the newest class member and to everyone's exercise response on the telemetry monitor. After twenty minutes, there's a switch to different machines. One woman wants to try the treadmill for the first time. The trainer gets her started and sticks close to assist with proper speed and form. The new gentleman is directed to a treadmill. He's shown how to get the tread started and slowly increased to his prescribed working pace and how to incorporate a long stride into each step. After six minutes, he reports a rate of perceived exertion of twelve—fairly light. Blood pressures are again taken and all are queried for RPE. "How hard are you working?" The woman trying the treadmill for the first time says she feels like she is working very hard. "I think I'm at a fifteen." The nurse, not particularly happy with the woman's blood pressure or pulse rate, stops the machine and has her sit down and drink a cup of water. Her vitals return to normal quickly, and she assures the staff that she is feeling fine, but she agrees that her treadmill speed should be reduced when she tries again during her mid-week class. Everyone heads to a separate room at the end of the gym for stretching and weight training.

The trainer, staying close to the new student, places her forearms and elbows against the wall and talks the group through a calf stretch. "Bend your left knee and move you right leg back behind your left. Keep your right leg straight, left knee bent, and both feet facing forward. Adjust your stance so that both heels remain on the floor. You should feel a comfortable stretch in your right calf. Hold the position without bouncing; remember that bouncing will cause the muscle to contract rather than expand. Now, we'll switch to the left leg and repeat the same motion." Standing sideways and gripping the handrail on the wall, they move into a quadriceps stretch, bringing the right knee up, pushing the leg backward, and grasping the right foot with a free hand. After several seconds, they lower their legs and turn around to do the same maneuver with the left leg. "Remember, you don't have to hold your foot," says the trainer. "If your leg cramps at that height, or you have to hunch over to reach your foot, just bring your leg up until you feel a comfortable stretch, or simply rest your knee on the seat of a chair." Exercisers continue to hold the bar and face the wall for toe raises—a slow roll up onto the toes, holding, and a roll back down until heels are on the floor. Away from the rail, but still standing, everyone puts first the right hand (with left hand supporting right elbow) back between the shoulder blades, holds and releases, and repeats on the other side for the triceps stretch. They complete a right and left side reach stretch by reaching one arm straight up, lowering it after several seconds, and then repeating with the other arm.

Handheld weights are doled out. "Three pounds?" questions the new gentleman. "I use to lift ten before my bypass surgery." The trainer suggests he start with three pounds to get acquainted with the wellness weight routine and to evaluate how he feels during

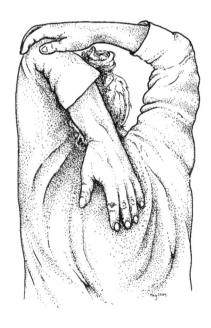

Triceps Stretch

each movement. "Why don't you try six repetitions to start. You'll increase that number over time," she assures him. Standing, the group begins with eight repetitions of a biceps curl. Holding a weight in each hand and with upper arms against their sides, everyone curls forearms toward the chest and back down. As they work, the trainer reviews proper weightlifting techniques. "Keep your knees slightly bent, and don't let you body sway." She encourages the class to exhale when they lift the weight and inhale when the weights are lowered. "I don't think I'll ever get this breathing down," says one woman. "It's the opposite of how I want to breathe." The trainer says, "Just make sure you're breathing. It's all about breathing versus holding your breath. Holding your breath elevates blood pressure." With arms down against sides,

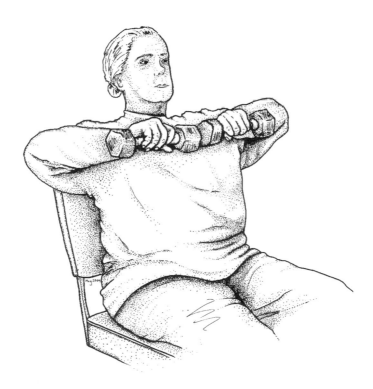

Upright Row

palms back, they slowly push the weights back and down for eight repetitions of the triceps extension.

The upright row is next. Holding the weights in front at the waist, lifting to the upper chest, and slowly lowering weights back down to waist level, they are on the forth repetition when the new gentleman chimes in. "Wow, even with only three pounds I can hardly do this one. It hurts my chest." The trainer has him stop. "You may experience chest discomfort in your incision area for quite some time. Four repetitions are enough for now, and on that particular lift, we can also think about changing to two-pound weights for a few weeks." As the class begins a military press, extending weights from shoulder height to arm's length above the head and back to shoulders, the same man has difficulty. He tries the press with two pounds and is much more comfortable.

Switching to lower body work, the trainer hands the three-pound weights back to the newcomer. "It's okay to accommodate your present health status with different weight sizes," she says. "The doing is more important than how much you're doing it with. As you move through the program, you will get stronger." Seated, and with hands supporting the two weights on the top of the right knee, the class lifts and lowers the weighted leg for four quadriceps raises. With foot on the floor and the weights still on the same knee, they raise just the heel off the floor and lower it back down for four heel raises. They repeat the two lifts with the left leg. Everyone's weight training RPE is determined, pulses and blood pressures are taken, and telemetry leads are removed. "Weight training is one of the best things that has happened to me," recalls Dick. "It makes me take better care of myself and be more concerned about my health."

Wednesday exercise is under way. Blood pressure and telemetry check-in procedure is complete. There's some discussion about a news report that was aired the night before regarding the pluses and minuses of drugs prescribed for lowering cholesterol. A class member donates a jazz CD recorded by her brother's band to play for the exercise period. The woman who had trouble on the treadmill on Monday gives it a go again. This time, she's well hydrated and working at a slightly lower rate of speed. She completes twelve

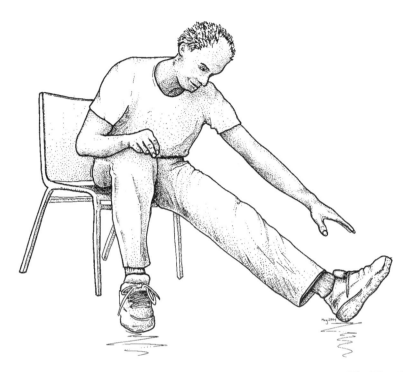

Toe-Touch

minutes with an RPE of fourteen—somewhat hard. The man who had his first day of exercise on Monday adds ten minutes to his treadmill time, works again on the NUSTEP, and gets instruction on using the elliptical machine. Working blood pressures are taken, and each exerciser moves comfortably through their workout, getting machines going and building up to prescribed speed and intensity. The staff chats with everybody individually and asks how hard they're working (the range is twelve to fourteen), while the group banter centers around recalling the names of the CD tunes playing in the background. Once the aerobic activity ends, they all move into the stretching/weight room.

The raised arm and shoulder is added to the calf, quadriceps, triceps, toe raise and side reach stretching routine. In this new motion, fingers are linked together, arms are raised overhead, and palms are up. A gentle pull from shoulders to fingertips is added. Seated, the class learns to do the toe-touch stretch. Extending the left leg out in front with heel on the floor and toes flexed, they move forward at the waist, reaching the left hand toward their toes. "Keep your torso straight, and just reach far enough to feel the stretch in you upper leg," says the trainer. "You don't actually have to touch your toes." They repeat on the right.

Staying seated, the group prepares for their Wednesday relaxation. Lights are dimmed. The room grows quiet. In the background, a CD plays the rolling and swishing of ocean waves. The trainer sits off to one side of the room. She begins to speak softly.

In the middle of each day, a few moments of attention to regular occurrences in nature can refresh and rejuvenate the mind and body. It can put life's ups and downs into perspective. Let's all relax into the ordinary.

Everyone, take a deep breath in ... exhale slowly.
Again, take in a deep, full breath ... and exhale fully.
Breathe in ... and clear your mind of yesterday's mistakes, today's to-do list, and the worries of tomorrow.
Exhale out ... and let go of any remaining concerns.
Close your eyes ... and imagine that you are on a beach.
You are the only person there.
You are sitting on a large piece of driftwood.
Your body is light ... your mind is quiet.
The gentle breeze of a thousand days past brushes your cheek and carries the sea aroma to your nostrils ... today you take time to notice ... feel the gentle breeze brush your cheek ... inhale the aroma of the sea.

Pause

One by one the waves of a thousand days past rumble to shore ... today you take time to notice ... hear them ... become attuned to their rhythm ... listen to the waves rumble and crash to shore ... listen to the waves clap back over the rocks and shells ... hear them swish out to sea ... breathe with them ... in and out.

Pause

Seagulls bob peacefully up and down on the gentle roll
of sea ... look today ... enjoy the simplicity ... watch the
seagulls bobbing up and down.

Pause

The sand of a thousand days sifts through your toes ...
today you notice ... feel the granules, warm on the bottoms
of your feet ... feel tiny grains of sand sift through your
toes.

Pause

Your seat of driftwood is rough ... notched and crevassed
with the buffeting of a thousand days ... and today you
notice ... run your hands along the knobs and depressions ...
feel the coarse ridges on your palms.

Pause

At your feet the grooved stones of a thousand days ... and
today you pick one up and fold it into your hand ... feel the
grooves of the stone as it twists and turns through your fingers.

Pause

Take a deep breath in ... exhale slowly and fully.
Take another breath in, a breath like those of a thousand
days ... and today you notice ... feel your lungs take in the
air ... exhale the breath out ... feel your body relax.

Pause

Open your eyes, as you've done a thousand times ... and
know that today is different ... today you've relaxed and
taken notice of the ordinary.

Everyone remains silent in the dim room. Blood pressures and
pulses are taken. Telemetry leads are removed. The gentleman
who joined the class on Monday says, "Thank you."

"You're very welcome," the trainer replies. "And all of you have a
great day."

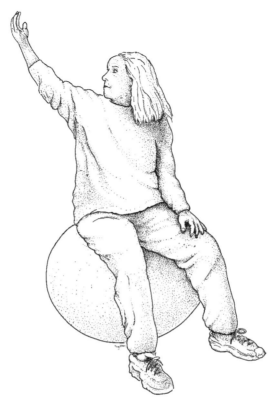

Oblique Stretch

It's the end of the week. The newest class member has become an old hand at applying his telemetry electrodes. Everyone is checked in and gets started with their five minute warm-up. This particular facility is on the ground floor of a community hospital. There is a large bird feeder (the brainchild of the wellness staff) right outside the gym windows, and a bevy of frenzied starlings are fluttering and cheeping to protest the large, black crow devouring their seeds. For some, today is a day for increasing aerobic workout time. As they work into the additional minutes, the nurse keeps a close eye on each of them on the telemetry computer screen. The trainer moves about the floor taking blood pressures and asking for RPE numbers. Helen, a wiry, energetic woman who is walking on a treadmill has increased her speed. She tells the trainer that she feels great. "Only my elbows are starting to hurt," she says. As the woman talks, the trainer quickly reduces her pace until the treadmill stops. The woman's discomfort begins to ease up. "Don't forget, Helen, for you, a first sign of angina is elbow pain," reminds the nurse who has arrived on the scene. "I just never seem to think of that," Helen replies, as she heads into the office for further evaluation.

During the stretching segment of the class, the trainer brings out one of the large inflated exercise balls. "Let me show you a fun oblique stretch." She lowers herself onto the ball in a seated position, rolling forward so that her feet are flat on the floor. Twisting slowly first to the right and then left, she demonstrates the move. She suggests that everybody place a chair on either side of their ball for added safety. "That way, if you lose your balance and roll to the side, you'll have the chair seat to lean on to stop your fall." Laughs and giggles abound as bodies weave and wobble onto the balls. Stretching side oblique muscles is eventually successful.

After eight repetitions of the now-familiar upright row, military press, and triceps extension, the trainer introduces two new lifts in a standing position. First is the triceps push-down. With both hands behind her head holding one weight, the trainer slowly pushes the weight straight up and back down. "Keep the weight behind your head, not over it, and don't forget to breathe," she says. "We'll do four repetitions. Remember, we cut reps in half for the first week or two of a new lift." She adds four lateral raises, lifting her arms and the weights out sideways away from her body

WEEK ONE OF CARDIAC EXERCISE— WHAT TO EXPECT

Your blood pressure will be checked and your workout will be monitored through telemetry. You will be introduced to aerobic equipment and learn how to put a physical value on the intensity of your workout by using the rate of perceived exertion (RPE) chart. You will begin a stretching routine and weight training with handheld weights. You may have a relaxation session.

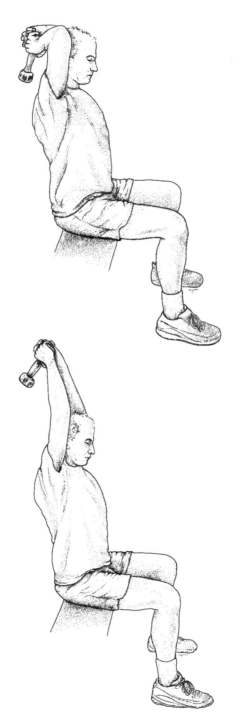

Triceps Push-Down

and up to shoulder height. "Keep your knees slightly bent, and if your arms start to tremble or shake, switch to a lighter weight. Raising the weights away from your body is a tough move. Using a lighter weight is okay." Seated, they do eight quadriceps raises and eight heel lifts with each leg. "I'm really amazed at the workout we can get just from hand weights," says one woman during the RPE and resting blood pressure check. "When you said we'd eventually be doing a total-body hand weight workout, I didn't get it."

Remembering the end of his first week in cardiac rehab, Dick says, "I felt I had found a perfect exercise situation. It forced me to get up, get going, and follow a routine. The personal interactions in Phase II and now in maintenance exercise have been fun and rewarding. Everybody is in these classes by choice, and their attitudes bespeak their desire to continue to enjoy life."

It is important for cardiac clients to made long-term commitments to exercise. "For some, it is the only way to maximize the heart muscles they have left," says Benner. "For others, it is part of risk reduction. When you look at the risk factors for cardiovascular disease, exercise affects them all positively."

7

EXERCISING FOR LIFE WITH DIABETES

DIABETES WELLNESS EXERCISE PHASE II

"The doors we open and close each day decide the lives we live."

OPENING THE DOOR to diabetes exercise is a healthy life decision. Diabetes is not running the show, you are, and you're headed in the direction of wellness.

A few years ago, a copilot for a large airline was thinking about testing to become a pilot. The requirements were stringent, and the exams would take weeks to complete. If he passed, he would have many new responsibilities. Unsure about proceeding, the man asked his father for advice. Without a moment's hesitation, the old gentleman replied, "Son, the pilot's chair is the only seat to be in." Taking over the piloting of your life isn't always easy. It, too, requires assuming new responsibilities, but for managing your illness and achieving the highest possible state of wellness, it's the only seat in the house. You are deciding how you will live, and behind the doors you open will be people and resources ready to honor and reinforce your commitment.

"Wellness has always made sense to me," says Mitzi Hazard, one of only a handful of physical therapists in the U.S. who is also a certified diabetes educator. As a college student working in a hospital physical therapy department, Hazard became involved with a fitness program for diabetics that had been created by one of the therapists. "I was fascinated at the number of people who were able to come off of their oral meds or decrease their dosages of insulin simply because they worked out at a moderate level three days a week." There's a personal side for Hazard, too. "My grandmother had diabetes, and I have the 'apple' shape, so I knew that one day I would as well."

Exercise is essential for people with diabetes. "It is clear the sedentary lifestyle is an epidemic in the country," says Hazard. "It is not coincidental that the rise in the number of television channels, reality shows, and computer games is matching the rate of diabetes and other diseases related to this lifestyle." Exercise is also the cheapest, easiest, and most physiologic way to manage diabetes. "The way I look at it, you can either take a handful of pills, which will each have their own nasty side effect and/or complication, or you can strap on a good pair of shoes and walk for thirty minutes." Along with the extensive list of benefits resulting from adhering to a regular workout, add for diabetics a possible decrease in vascular inflammation (an increasingly recognized problem in diabetes and heart disease), a decrease in blood sugar levels, increased insulin sensitivity, and improved glucose tolerance. Also, if exercise is regular and consistent, it removes another variable in things that affect blood glucose.

One of the first things Hazard does in preparing a client's exercise prescription is look at their feet and shoes. "I make sure that their shoes are in good shape and supportive for their foot type, and then I test their sensation. Neuropathy (loss of or altered sensation) does not preclude starting an exercise program, but it makes us approach it a little more carefully." The next step is to sort out what, if any, chronic complications of diabetes exist. Heart and cerebrovascular disease, neuropathy, retinopathy and/or nephropathy may be evident. "To an extent, the complications dictate which exercise precautions must be taken, says Hazard. "Anyone embarking on a formal exercise program should undergo a thorough medical evaluation that includes risk evaluation of micro and macrovascular complications. Before beginning exercises with me, I request a prescription from their doctor which stipulates parameters for heart rate, blood pressure, and oxygen saturation, if that is appropriate to their disease process." As part of the interview and assessment, Hazard has a discussion with her clients regarding their expectations, goals, type of exercise they are willing to do, and time of day they are most likely to do it. A person's blood glucose control is considered in the design of the diabetic's workout formula. "If their numbers are not within range, we do not want to start a formal exercise program until that happens. Regular exercise will initially upset the balance as we try to get energy expenditure and energy intake in balance. I want to make sure that their blood glucose excursions are as predictable as possible."

In the wellness program, blood glucose will be checked and documented pre-and post-workout. "The reason is to make sure that they are safe to exercise and so that the client is aware of how exercise affects their blood glucose," says Hazard. "When they are new to exercise, I also ask them to step up their at-home monitoring, since exercise is so effective at continuing to decrease blood glucose levels for twelve to seventy-two hours later." As a general rule, the blood glucose ranges for safe exercise are a minimum of 100mg/dL and a maximum of 300 for people who are not on insulin. For those who are on insulin, the general rule maximum is 240.

As with blood glucose, blood pressure and heart rate will be noted pre-and post-exercise. During each workout, your activity and vitals will be checked and recorded. Measurements can include heart rate, blood pressure, oxygen saturations for anyone with pulmonary issues, equipment used and amount of time, warm-up and working speed, power output (WATTS), metabolic equivalents (METS), size of dumbbells used for weightlifting, and rate of perceived exertion (RPE). Rate of perceived exertion is defined by using the RPE chart (see inside covers). The chart will help you assign a value to your workout. It will have numbers on one side and descriptions of physical exertion levels on the other: legs heavy, muscles a little tired, getting hard to talk, fourteen—somewhat hard. Medically pertinent information that you discuss with the nurse or other facilitators will also be posted. Staff notes will be recorded.

In regard to a target heart rate, Hazard says, "What I want to know most is what heart rate/blood pressure levels they should not exceed. Then I have them use the perceived exertion scale in terms of intensity of exercise. It (RPE) is so functional, and people are generally much less frustrated than when trying to teach them how to measure their heart rate and where they should be for a target. It gives them a certain measure of freedom and independence that I like. For me, it is all about them making it on their own."

LET'S SPEND A WEEK in diabetes wellness exercise. There will be similarities and differences from program to program, but by coming along on this excursion you'll get a jump-start on the basics. This particular course consists of one-hour sessions held three times a week.

This is the first day of exercise for everyone in the class. The procession into the workout area is slow. Folks do a quick and cautious visual sweep of the gym and the equipment. Seats are taken, and the diabetes wellness nurse checks and records blood pressures and pulses. Everyone is interested in their numbers. "That sure is lower than the readings I get in my doc's office. I guess I'm calmer here," shares one man. Blood glucose readings are next. The nurse assists those who are new to using a glucose monitor. Others do their own testing. One person's sugar is high, but within a safe range for exercise.

It's time to get to work. On the advice of the nurse, two gentlemen with evidence of neuropathy settle in on the recumbent bikes. She shows them the adjustment techniques particular to the machines and how to get started at an easy five-minute warm-up speed. Two other people learn the safe use of treadmills. "The last time I was on one of these treadmill things, it was for my heart test," says one woman. "I was so nervous it made me sick, but I'm feeling pretty comfortable today." Stationary bikes hum, and a fellow is shown how to use the elliptical machine. With all exercisers past warm-up, a personal trainer circulates around the gym, defines the rate of perceived exertion (RPE) chart to each person, and reinforces how to put a value on the intensity of their workout. "Think about how hard you're working. How do you feel? Are you legs tired? Are you short of breath? Or, would you say you have no real discomfort and feel you're working in the fairly light range, say, eleven or twelve?" Speeds are slowly increased. After a few minutes at their faster pace, all are asked to identify their RPE. "How hard do you think you are working?" In accordance with responses, slight increases or decreases in speed are made. On this first day, most people work out on the initial machine for fifteen minutes, get a pulse check, and, with staff direction, move on to a different exercise. Each new user sees a demonstration of correct operation of recumbent and stationary bikes, treadmills, and the elliptical machine. One of the men with neuropathy learns the ins and outs of cranking the hand cycle, the other is shown how to use the NUSTEP recumbent with movable handles that will give him some upper body work. Another gentleman gets started on a rower. "Just like in the good old days with my dad on Culver's Lake," he says. "Except then I could row for hours." RPE is again asked of each person. "How hard are you working?" The fellow who has been on the rower for seven minutes says twenty. "Just kidding," he adds. "But fifteen is no joke. This is tough work." After a cool down and hydrating with water, it's on to stretching and weights.

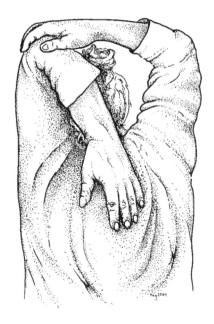

Triceps Stretch

The trainer has each exerciser stand behind a chair, and guides them into a quadriceps stretch. Holding the back of their chair with their left hand, they all bring the right knee up, push the right leg back, and grasp the right foot with the right hand. They learn to move slowly into the stretch, hold, and move back out. "If you feel any cramping, let go of your foot, and move you leg down lower," the trainer advises. "Or, you can just rest your knee on the chair seat." With both hands gripping the back of the chair, the group begins toe raises: a slow roll up onto the toes, holding, and rolling back down to heels on the floor. Demonstrating a standing lunge, the trainer shows the class the difference between static and ballistic stretching. She places her left leg in front of the right in a stance wide enough to situate her left knee over left toes. Both feet are pointing forward and heels are on the floor. Leaning into the stretch, she places her hands on her forward knee. "Always do a static stretch. Go into the position and hold it for fifteen seconds or so," she says. "Ballistic stretching involves bouncing (she demonstrates with a few bounces), and that can contract your muscles rather than expand them." Seated, the class executes a triceps stretch by putting the left hand (with right hand supporting left elbow) back between the shoulder blades and holding. After repeating on the other side, they segue into a foot point and flex. Extending one leg out and off the floor, toes are pointed toward the far wall. After a few seconds in that position, and with leg still off the floor, the foot is flexed toward the ceiling and held. The move is repeated with the other leg.

Handheld weights are doled out. Remaining seated, the class begins a few upper body lifts. With a weight in each hand and upper arms against their sides, everyone curls forearms toward the chest and back down to complete six biceps curls. For six triceps extensions, they place arms down against sides, with palms facing back, and slowly push the weights back and down again. Raising their shoulders up to their ears and back down, everyone completes six shoulder shrugs. Six military presses follow, with everyone extending the weights from shoulder height to arm's length above the head and back down to shoulders. "Always try and exhale on the exertive portion of the lift and inhale as you lower the weights," the trainer says. "Most importantly, don't hold your breath. It elevates your blood pressure." The class jokes through the routine with faux moans and groans. After weights, pulses are taken and blood glucose is rechecked. In each case, the numbers are lower than they had been at the beginning of class. "Wow," comments the gentleman who originally had a high glucose reading. "With just that little bit of exercise my sugar is down."

Diabetes client Harriet remembers her first day of Phase II exercise. "It was the way the 'first' of anything would be—uncertainty about who would be in the class, as well as not knowing about all of the machines."

Day two of exercise starts out just like the first—blood pressures, pulses, and blood glucose numbers. There is lively banter about the aftermath of the first day's workout.

"My legs definitely knew I did something different," says one woman.

"My whole body knew," another woman chimes in. "But I sure felt good for having done it."

The diabetes nurse is today's solo class facilitator. She invites everyone to head to the machines. One person easily adjusts the height of his bicycle seat, another remembers her treadmill warm-up speed and how to get the machine going. Everyone is individually checked during start-up, and exercise is underway. Use of the RPE chart to place a value on each workout is reinforced. On this day, some folks are oriented to new machines that they can incorporate into their pattern of aerobic work. The two men who have neuropathy and are avoiding extended weight-bearing work stick to the recumbent bicycles and hand cycle. Each exerciser completes thirty-five minutes of training.

After the quadriceps stretch, toe raise and lunge, two new standing stretches are added: arm circles, raising both arms out from the sides away from the body to shoulder height, and circling slowly one way and then the other, and head leans, rolling and holding the head sideways first toward the left and then to the right.

Lights are dimmed, and the soft sounds of violin and flute emanate from a CD player in the back of the room. The nurse pulls all the chairs into a circle, and everyone takes a seat for the group's first relaxation session.

"Here's a fun and simple way to relax and get to know a little bit about each other," the nurse says. "I like to call it a sharing circle. We all have favorite places. Your favorite place may be a spot that you visit regularly, or it may be a memory: a place for enjoyment, relaxation, perhaps solitude. Let's go around the circle, and share special places." The woman to the right of the nurse jumps in.

"I love to go to the ocean." Two others in the class agree.

"Give me a boat, a fishing pole, and a lake any day," says one of the men. "Just like when I was a kid with my dad on Culver's Lake."

Another gentleman adds, "I always liked to go for walks in the woods. It really got me in touch with nature. I should probably start doing that again." One of the two remaining group members concurs. The other says, "I could be happy in any one of those places as long as there were no phones, fax machines, or people."

The nurse smiles, "I'm with you. So, let's go on a walk to favorite places. Get comfortable in your seats. Close your eyes, and begin to inhale and exhale slowly. Relax into your breathing. With each inhale, you let go of any interfering thoughts. With each exhale, your body gets lighter and lighter. Inhale, clear you mind ... exhale, light and easy into the moment." Her voice lowers. She speaks slowly.

> Your walk begins on a sandy, narrow path ... on either side, delicate beach grass sways back and forth in the gentle breeze. The path leads to an expanse of beach ... white sand dotted with shells and nestling gulls is warm beneath your feet ... ocean waves rumble to shore ... pulling and whispering back into themselves ... the white sail of a sloop waves on the horizon. Take in this place ... inhale the sights, sounds, the smells of the sea ... exhale ... your body is light ... you are free of tension. If this is your favorite place, stay for a while and continue to relax.
>
> If you wish to continue your walk, move back along the sandy, narrow path, away from the sea. A new path lies before you ... fragrant, towering pine trees line either side ... their rich aroma permeates the air. The path leads into thick,

lush woods ... dried leaves and brittle twigs crunch and snap underfoot ... the air is crisp and clean ... the music of birds drifts through twisted branches ... a woodpecker drills a nesting place in the bark of a tree ... yellow buttercups poke through blades of emerald grass. Take in this place ... inhale the sights, sounds, and aromas of the woods ... exhale ... your body is light ... you are free of tension. If this is your favorite place, feel free to stay and continue to relax here.

To continue, walk further along the wooded trail to the clearing just ahead. The aqua lake is still ... a fresh-water duck glides silently across the surface ... four tiny, fury ducklings paddle behind ... smoke circles from the chimney of a small log cabin ... the scent of burning wood is sweet and strong ... reflections of trees ripple in the water ... across the lake, a rowboat bobs in front of the small cove ... a figure in the boat is silhouetted against the rising sun ... crickets are chirping. Take in this place ... inhale the sights, sounds, scents of the lake ... exhale ... your body is light ... you are free of tension.

Pause

Begin, now, to come back from your excursion ... breathe easily in ... and slowly out. Open your eyes ... breathe easily in ... and slowly out. Stretch your arms overhead, and continue easy breathing. Stretch your legs out, continue easy breathing. Slowly, lower your arms, and relax your legs. Inhale deeply ... exhale fully. Come back into the group dynamic, and take the memory of your favorite place with you into the rest of the day.

The class is surprised and pleased with their low resting pulse. Blood sugars are all within normal limits. "I always do feel better after a trip to the coast," says one woman. "Yeah, I know what you mean," one of the men adds. "I think it's time for me to plan a fishing trip."

There's a hint of confidence on the third day of exercise. People get right into the swing of things, all doing their blood glucose testing, others checking their own pulses. They get into their workout unassisted and get started on warm-up. The session is alive with chatter and jokes, and when asked how hard they're working, all are quick with an RPE number. There's a natural flow from machine to machine, as exercisers move comfortably about the gym. They are all encouraged to increase aerobic workout time an additional ten minutes. No moans or groans today, and everyone is pleased with their aerobic achievements. "I've been waiting all week to email my son," shares one woman. "He'll never believe I've come this far and that I'm planning to continue."

The full stretching routine is completed with no bouncing. A raised arm and shoulder move is added. For this, fingers are linked together and arms are raised overhead, palms up, pulling the stretch from shoulders to fingertips.

Six repetitions of a seated upright row are included in the weightlifting. These are accomplished by holding the weights in

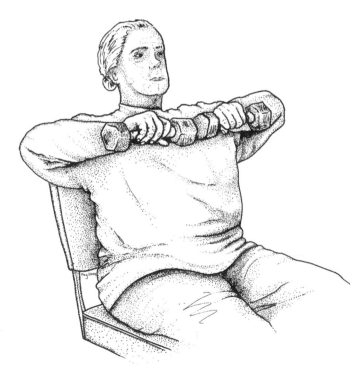

Upright Row

front at the waist, lifting them to the upper chest, and moving them slowly back down to waist level. Six seated lateral raises are added, too. The weights are positioned at sides and arms are slowly raised out away from the body to shoulder level. "Don't forget to breathe when you lift," the trainer reminds them, "Exhale on the lift or exertive portion, and inhale when the weights are lowered. Or, just breathe. If this lateral raise seems hard, and your arm muscles start to quiver, use lighter weights. It's okay to reduce weight size on lifts that are difficult." They continue with six repetitions of the biceps curl, triceps extension, military press, and shoulder shrug.

"The first week of class just solidified my feelings that this was a good choice for me," says Harriet. "Being part of the class guaranteed that I would actually do the exercises rather than fudge and just gallop through them if I were to do them at home. Besides, the group of fellow exercisers was very congenial, and I enjoyed the company."

The beginning of diabetes exercise kicks off your decision to pursue a new personal health standard and a higher quality of life. You've taken control. Congratulate yourself. You are in the pilot's seat, and it's the only seat in the house.

It is important for diabetes clients to make long-term commitments to exercise. "It is one of the most important weapons in their anti-diabetes arsenal," says Hazard. "It should be as important

WEEK ONE OF DIABETES EXERCISE— WHAT TO EXPECT

You will have blood pressure, pulse, and blood glucose testing. You will be introduced to aerobic equipment. You will learn how to use the rate of perceived exertion (RPE) chart to put a personal physical value on the intensity of your workout. You will begin a stretching routine and weight training with handheld weights. A relaxation session may be held.

as brushing teeth. It is an essential tool that helps to not only manage their disease process, but it staves off heart disease and some of the other nasty complications of diabetes. Exercise is also important because one of the biggest struggles in type 2 diabetes is weight management. Successful and long-term weight management requires a level of physical activity." Harriet, who faithfully sets aside time to continue to exercise in a wellness maintenance program, sums it up. "The overall experience has been better than anticipated. I find I am in much better physical condition than I was before. I walk better and have more stamina. All in all, it is quite a success."

Hazard has one of the best reasons for diabetics to stick to a fitness plan. "Regular exercise will bring your body as close as it will ever be to not knowing it has diabetes."

It is important to note that not all wellness programs offer phase II exercise to diabetes clients. If that is the case, with a referral from your physician, your diabetes coordinator can refer you directly into wellness maintenance if it is available, or work with you to design a safe and effective workout for use in a community gym, exercise class, or as an undertaking to do on you own.

———————

8

EXERCISING FOR LIFE WITH COPD

PULMONARY WELLNESS EXERCISE PHASE II

"To overcome difficulties is to experience the full delight of existence."

SHE BOUGHT A THIRTY-FOUR-FOOT sloop and sailed the boat on her own from Hawaii to Washington State. After single-handing back to Hawaii, she and a friend sailed around the world. She settled in the Pacific Northwest and wrote sailing articles, penned her first book, started a condiment business, and was diagnosed with lung disease. Her name was Annie, and COPD didn't stand in her way. With oxygen tank in tow, she continued her business, worked on a second book, did a little traveling, started taking art classes, and participated in wellness exercise. Annie *did* overcome her difficulties. She faced her illness and forged ahead. She continued to grow and experience her own existence with full delight, while adding humor, joy, and inspiration to the lives of those around her.

Like Annie, you are overcoming difficulties. The idea of getting started in an exercise program may seem incompatible with being short of breath or having to tote an oxygen tank, but you will find the safeguarded wellness training design congruous with a number of pulmonary issues. Bill, a former smoker and graduate of pulmonary Phase II, regularly attends maintenance exercise. Bill uses a walker and portable oxygen equipment and says he never thought about any planned exercise before joining pulmonary rehabilitation. "I had to do something or wind up in a nursing home." You have to do something, too.

As part of determining your individual workout schedule,

starting a pulmonary program will involve fitness testing. "We do a six-minute walk test," says registered respiratory therapist Katherine Riddle. "We try and do it at the initial evaluation, but it depends on whether or not we feel they're stable enough for it. That (the test) gives the exercise physiologist a baseline to see how blood saturation levels respond to exercise and also how their body as a whole responds." For Riddle's pulmonary clients, a wellness facility seventy-five-foot track is used to conduct a low-grade walk test. "Not everyone is able to go on a treadmill, and if they are not used to being on a treadmill there's too much of a learning adjustment going on." The client walks the track at his or her own speed and is given an introduction to the rate of perceived exertion (RPE) and rate of perceived dyspnea (RPD) charts that will help them assign a value to the intensity of the activity and to their breathing. These charts have numbers on one side and descriptions of physical exertion and breathing levels on the other. An example of a physical evaluation would be: legs feeling heavy, muscles a little tired, difficult to talk, fourteen—somewhat hard. The same concept is used to appraise breathing: fairly easy to breathe—eleven. "Not everyone is able to walk for a total of six minutes," says Riddle. "We encourage them to pace themselves. It's actually their first lesson in self-pacing, and if I'm going to start them on a treadmill at their first exercise visit, it gives me a chance to look at their gait and lets me see what speed would be appropriate for them. Also, if there are any ailments going on, whether in their back or any of their joints, I can determine what other modality would be appropriate for them to start out on." Coming up with a baseline exercise prescription may take longer than the initial six-minute walk test. "There can be a lot of fear and anxiety. Some patients are afraid to really push themselves, so it might take a couple of weeks to figure out their baseline and appropriate intensity level," says Riddle. If that is the case, a non-weight-bearing machine that supports the body and allows the patient to exercise arms and legs while in a sitting position will be used at first. The intensity will be very low. "I want them to be able to maintain their sats (oxygen saturations) at ninety percent or above before I get them up and walking." If you have not had a pulmonary function test or electrocardiogram (EKG) within six months, those tests may be done the day of your initial assessment, prior to the intake interview.

During your exercise sessions, a pulse oximeter will be used to monitor your oxygen saturation (the percent of hemoglobin saturated with oxygen). A probe attached to a small computerized unit will be placed on your fingertip or ear lobe. The computer will display the percent of oxygen saturation and pulse rate. One reason to use the oximeter is to help you understand that shortness of breath is a valid symptom. "For a lot of people, we're actually showing them that, yes, with that shortness of breath there is a drop in oxygen level," says Riddle. "Hence, that helps them to learn how to self-pace based on their breathing." Some COPD patients will show a drop in oxygen saturation during exercise and not experience shortness of breath. Seeing the low number will help them recognize other symptoms that may signal the drop. "A lot of people who don't say they're short of breath will tell us that their legs feel really tired, or that they feel tired," says Riddle. "We try and help them correlate some physical symptom as their guide so that when they're out in the real world they know they need to slow down, do their purse-lip breathing or belly breathing, or whatever technique works for them to help them recover. We try hard to figure out what is the symptom that we can relate to the number so that we can keep you safe."

You will likely be given an exercise target heart rate of sixty to eighty percent of maximum. "It's not necessary to work over eighty percent," says exercise physiologist Mary Price. "I want people to understand that you don't have to kill yourself and be out there training like your elite athletes do to acquire a healthy fitness level." Price encourages going for the low end of the target. "Research has shown that working at sixty percent, you're going to gain all the physiological benefits of exercise."

At the beginning of each class, initial blood pressure, resting pulse, oxygen saturation, and weight will be documented. During each workout, your activity and vitals will be recorded. This can include heart rate, blood pressure, oxygen saturation, equipment used and amount of time, warm-up and working speed, power output (WATTS), metabolic equivalents (METS), size of dumbbells used for weightlifting, rate of perceived exertion (RPE), and rate of perceived dyspnea (RPD) (see inside covers). Medically pertinent information discussed with the nurse or other facilitators will also be posted. Staff notes will be recorded.

In the pulmonary education classes, you will learn better breathing techniques. These new skills will come in handy during the exercise sessions. Purse-lip breathing can help in recovering from shortness of breath and can also increase oxygen saturation levels. Says Riddle, "When someone drops their sats and I'm standing there watching and I say let me see your purse-lip breathing, within three to five purse-lip breaths they can watch their oxygen level climb. Then we teach it as a preventative. You look at what you're going to do and if it's going to be exertive, start your purse-lip breathing as you go into it." Blowing out slowly through pursed lips decelerates exhalation. It also creates back pressure that opens the upper airways so more air is exhaled. "We call it 'Smell the roses, blow out the candle,' " adds Riddle. "They're breathing in through their nose and then blowing out as if they're blowing out a candle." As you learn to think about breathing from the belly, you can fill your lungs more effectively. It also helps with stress. "When people are in an anxious or stressed state, they begin purse-lip breathing and then from that they go into belly breathing, and it's incredible how that can just slow and calm things down."

LET'S SPEND A WEEK in pulmonary wellness exercise. There will be similarities and differences from program to program, but by coming along on this excursion you'll get a jump-start on the basics. This particular course consists of one-hour classes held three times a week.

Of the six people who arrive for Monday afternoon pulmonary exercise, four are using portable oxygen. They are all a few weeks into the program, and all are fifteen minutes early for class. "We like to have a chance to sit a bit before exercise to be sure our oxygen numbers are above ninety," says one of the women. They're soon weighing-in on the scale. The nurse and personal trainer arrive and engage each client in a friendly health query and general conversation as resting blood pressures and pulse oximetry numbers are noted. The results, along with each person's weight, are entered into the computer.

As people move to the stationary bicycles, treadmills, and recumbent bikes, a seventh class member, also on oxygen, arrives in a wheelchair. With everyone settled into their five-minute warm-up, the nurse checks-in the man in the wheelchair and heads him toward a hand cycle that is secured to a tabletop. With his wheelchair situated in front of the hand cycle, he grips the handlebars, and starts a slow rotational arm movement. After three minutes, the nurse checks his oxygen saturation level. He's at ninety-two. Another three minutes and he's dropped to eighty-six. He says his RPD feels like thirteen—somewhat short of breath. RPE is somewhat hard, also thirteen. After a blood pressure check, he wants to continue for another few minutes, but the nurse has him stop at six minutes and drink a cup of water. "Don't forget," she says. "Last week you only did three minutes before your sats dropped below ninety. You are improving."

Twenty minutes into the workout, the others in the class have had blood pressures taken, oxygen saturations checked, and have evaluated their RPE and RPD. Re-hydrated, everyone heads to a different machine; those who started on the stationary bikes switch to treadmills, another person moves to the hand cycle, and one fellow climbs on the rower. The man in the wheelchair is using a walker to take a few steps around the gym. The nurse keeps watch on his oxygen saturation. A woman on a treadmill increases her speed and also adds a slight incline to the workout. After a few minutes, her oxygen is down to eight-nine. "It's better to stick to one increase at a time," says the trainer. "Let's try doing away with the incline and see what happens." It isn't long before she's up to ninety-two. A few people move on to get in some time on a third machine. Others go to the weight room to begin stretching.

With the entire group together in the weight room, the trainer leads them through a series of seated stretches. They start with head leans, rolling the head sideways first toward the left shoulder and then to the right shoulder, holding each position for several seconds. Placing the right hand on the upper back between the shoulder blades and using the left to push gently on the right elbow, a triceps stretch is carried out, reversed, and repeated, followed by everybody leaning forward from the waist for toe touches. For this position, they reach the right arm toward an extended right foot. Heel is on the floor, toes are flexed. After about twelve seconds, this is repeated with the left arm and foot. "Remember, you don't have to actually touch your toes," reminds the trainer. "Just keep your torso straight and lean toward your foot until you feel a comfortable stretch in you leg." Slow, wide arm circles are next, first one way, then the other. Now, with both hands on right hamstring muscle on the backside of the upper leg, they lift the right knee toward the chest, hold, and lower for a single knee to chest stretch. Switching hands to left hamstring, the left knee is raised toward the chest and down. "Here's a new one called point

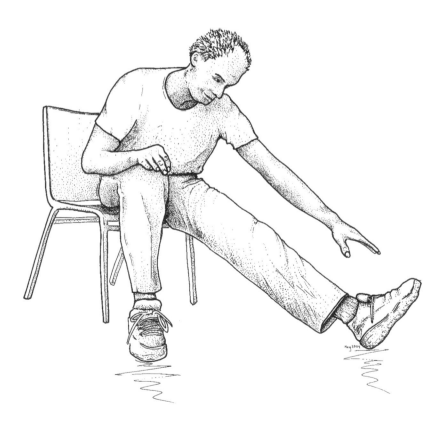

Toe Touch

and flex." The trainer demonstrates, and folks follow along. One leg is extended out and up, off the floor. Toes are pointed toward the far wall. After a few seconds, with leg still extended and off the floor, the foot is flexed toward the body so toes are pointing to the ceiling. The stretch is repeated with the other leg. "Wow! Can I ever feel that behind my knee," says one woman.

Handheld weights are given out for seated weight training. The trainer suggests they increase their workout. "We've been doing six repetitions of each lift for a few weeks. Let's shoot for eight today, but if you have any discomfort, I want you to stop." Holding a weight in each hand and with upper arms against their sides, everyone curls forearms toward the chest and back down for eight biceps curls. For the triceps extensions, arms are down against

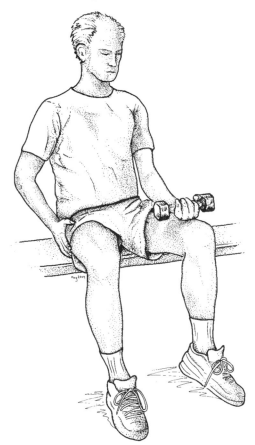

Quadriceps Raises

sides, palms are facing back, and the weights are slowly pushed back and down again. They continue with the military press, extending weights from shoulder level to arm's length above the head and back down to shoulders. "Don't forget to breathe," reminds the trainer. "No holding your breath." Two people stop at six presses. The gentleman in the wheelchair gets to eight. "Well, I couldn't have done that a few weeks ago," he says. Holding the weights in front at the waist, lifting to upper chest and slowly back down, eight upright rows are completed. Using two hands to support both weights on the top of the right knee, quadriceps raises are executed by lifting the weighted leg up and down for eight repetitions. The same lift is done with the left leg. RPE and RPD assessments are noted. As the trainer begins taking resting blood pressures and final oxygen saturations, the nurse arrives with balloons and a diploma. A class member has completed all of his education and exercise classes. He is graduating from the Phase II pulmonary program. Kudos and a round of applause follow. "I won't be far away," he says. "I'm planning on joining maintenance exercise."

A driving rain doesn't deter the group from attending their Wednesday afternoon class. Check-in is energetic as the choice of workout music is debated. A CD of Broadway show tunes is the winner. Machines start to hum with the sounds of warm-up. The fellow in the wheelchair feels good after five minutes working his upper body on the hand cycle. His RPE and RPD are both fairly light at eleven and oxygen saturation a reasonably good ninety-two. He manages to complete three more minutes with good numbers. Everyone remains stable and active throughout the aerobic segment of exercise.

Seated, the class completes head leans, toe touches, and a triceps stretch. The room lights are dimmed in preparation for Wednesday's relaxation.

The trainer sits in front of the group. "Chronic illness challenges you to face, accept, and move through physical and emotional upheaval," she says. "Successful management of chronic illness involves change. Today's relaxation session is about change. All you have to do is get comfortable and listen to a story." She unfolds a yellowed, dog-eared magazine article and begins to read.

It was day three—early morning. A low fog draped across the bay, closing in on the barking otters. The ferry glided from the dock and disappeared into the mist. In the orchard on the side of the house, an elegant doe and her two spotted fawns munched apples that had fallen from the trees. The late October air numbed my bare feet, but it was hard to move from the porch. The outside distractions were welcomed.

Inside, the coffeepot grumbled through its perk cycle, while the ancient furnace sputtered and groaned warmth up to the icy kitchen. The toaster sprung. I poked the crisp bagel out and slathered it with cream cheese. It was his favorite breakfast. The popping toaster and squeaking cheese container would always bring him to the kitchen, but not today. I opened a yogurt container (another of his favorites) and shook the cookie jar. He did not come.

Except to drink some water and make hasty trips to the yard to relieve his ballooning innards, Sunny, my cocker spaniel companion of ten years, had kept his round body wedged in the small space behind the blue, overstuffed rocking chair. His beige, freckled face and black nose stayed tightly pushed into the seam of the wall at the far end of the living room. The ribbons of silky hair on his long ears rippled down to the floor, blending with the tan carpet. His stubby tail wagged when his name was mentioned, but the rest of him remained firm. Just two weeks before, during his yearly checkup, the veterinarian had said, "This is the happiest dog I know," but Sunny wasn't happy any more. It was Wednesday—the start of day three—and Sunny was still in the corner.

The plea had come via email. A good friend in Seattle was divorcing. She would barely be able to manage her two children. I was the only one she trusted. Would I *PLEASE* take her young dog? Giving little thought to the consequences of adopting my friend's pet, in the early morning hours of the previous Monday I had headed to the city.

Fudge pop eyes twinkled through a snowy coat. Pointed, pink-lined ears stood at attention. A curious black nose sniffed my hand. Fifteen pounds of sweet-smelling white fur plopped into my lap. A slow, wet tongue on my cheek sealed the transaction.

"His name is Brodie, he's a West Highland terrier, almost a year old, and I just can't thank you enough," said my friend through hugs and tears.

"Ooh, how cute."

"Is it a boy or girl?"

"What's its name?"

"Can we pet him?"

The ferry from Seattle to Bainbridge Island was overflowing with kids—curious, bouncy, exuberant kids—on my lap, on my toes, on the floor with the dog. Brodie rolled over for belly pats. "Another happy pup," I sighed with relief.

The hour-long ride home from Bainbridge was perfect. Brodie curled in the front passenger seat of the Jeep and slept. I stroked him periodically, but there was no sound, and only the movement of easy breathing. In the days to come I would consider the possibility that my "friend" had slipped Brodie a Valium before our introduction in Seattle.

Once home, he tore into the house. He ran through the kitchen, up the stairs, through each of the bedrooms, back downstairs for a dash through my office, and two loops around the living room. Back in the kitchen, he took a hearty drink from the water bowl and ran the course again. He whirled in a circle, chasing his tail. He leapt onto the couch and onto the floor. He skidded back to the kitchen and came to a crashing halt against Sunny, who wobbled and staggered out of peaceful sleep.

Brodie sniffed wildly, from Sunny's wet nose to frozen tail. He nipped, jumped on and off Sunny's shivering body, and ran back and forth, challenging the stupefied cocker to chase. He yapped and snorted in Sunny's face and pawed at his trembling jowls. Except for a puzzled glance at me, the commotion immobilized the normally mellow old dog. After a slow recovery from paralysis, Sunny lumbered through the living room. He heaved his old body into position. The fireplace andirons rattled and clanked. Whining morosely, he settled in behind the rocker. And now, on day three, Sunny remained in the corner.

The transition had been no less traumatic for Brodie. Twice he had tumbled into the bathtub while trying to escape the wrath of my spitting cat. Fleeing the loud whir of the vacuum, he had gotten locked in a closet and relieved his angst by peeing on my new walking shoes. Out in the yard, the grazing deer sent him into a frenzy of hysterical running and earsplitting barking that rattled the neighborhood. And several times a day, Brodie had gone to the far corner of the living room to yap his high-pitched Westie yap at Sunny's stationary rump. Now, on the morning of day three I, too, was frazzled, and folded into the couch pillows for a good cry. I had decided my bawling would kickoff an extended period of remorse and feeling sorry for myself.

Two warm, sloppy tongues began lapping my cheeks. Brodie nested on the top of my head, peering down into my face. His tail vibrated against the lamp on the side table. Sunny planted himself in front of me and nudged my body, first with one paw and then the other. I looked into two wise and mysterious faces. *They knew* I was heading for some serious wallowing. *I knew* what they were communicating. With the beasts orchestrating the enlightenment of the "higher" animal, I scrubbed the long agenda of self-pity and followed their lead to get on with life. Going to the dogs, I began critter observation.

Over the course of the next few days, we became a positive, functioning pack. Sunny, who loved food more than anything, was given first licks from the yogurt container and the first piece of bagel. Little Brodie waited his turn. Brodie, who loved play more than anything, got first pick of any new chew toys. Sunny claimed the remaining rawhide. Brodie's day required at least one mad run from room to room, and thundering across the porch, now in fearless pursuit of the cat. During these activities, Sunny retired to the safety of the couch and I played an Enya CD. Sunny's needs included ear stroking from all visitors, and naps in sunbeams. To accommodate, Brody moved in behind Sunny for petting, and slept in the thinnest portions of sunlight. Out on the beach, Brodie displayed the most exuberance. Running free, chasing gulls, he'd disappear into clouds of sand, but always ran mightily back to Sunny and me when his distance became too great. His return would be rewarded with a leg or two of fresh crab Sunny had fished out.

In a short time, they had adapted well. The precarious beginnings of their relationship behind them, the dogs had rallied, sassy and happy, forgiving and forgetting. I was in awe of their hasty return to balance under the duress of change. While I had mustered the maturity to adapt to life with two dogs without prolonged pouting, I knew I was still laden with years of conditioning in the human tangle of "why me" indulgences. I doubted my ongoing ability to recoup quickly and move assuredly through adversity. I thought, perhaps, I'd spend a few days in the corner.

The room buzzes with pet tales and dialogue on change. Blood pressures are well within normal limits, and oxygen above ninety is unanimous. The class moves slowly toward the door, lingering over chuckles and conversation.

It's the last day of pulmonary exercise for the week. Check-in is routine for everyone, and the class gets started. One woman arrives late and mentions that she's been experiencing more shortness of breath than usual. The nurse listens to the woman's lungs and the two go into the nurse's office. The personal trainer works with the exercisers. Travel and RV campers are the topics of conversation. By the end of the aerobic segment, everyone has added five minutes to their workout, and vitals have remained within normal limits. The client having breathing problems is heading to her doctor's office for further evaluation.

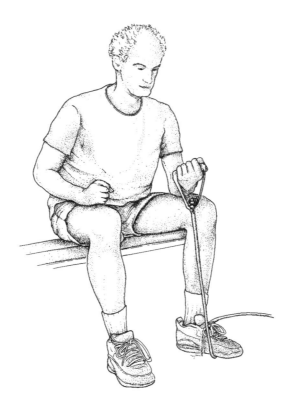

Wrist Curl

In the weight room, the trainer places her forearms and elbows against a wall and demonstrates a calf stretch. "Lean into the wall, bend the left knee, and move the right leg behind the left. Keep the right leg straight and left knee bent. Be sure both feet are facing forward and both heels are on the floor. You'll feel a comfortable stretch in the right calf." Taking a little time to get into position and fix foot direction, the class follows, holds the position for ten seconds, and changes sides. Toe touch, triceps, point and flex seated stretching is uniform and smooth. Each movement is held for several seconds with no bouncing. The trainer introduces wrist curls with resistance bands and hand weights. Seated, and with a hand in each handle of a resistance band, the trainer drops the center of the tubing to the floor and places her feet on top to hold it secure. With forearms on her lap (on quadriceps muscles) and while holding the handles of the band, she curls her wrists forward and down. After several repetitions, she puts the band aside, and switches to weights to do the same wrist movement. The class follows suit for four repetitions of each. Next, they complete eight reps of familiar weight lifts: upright rows, biceps curls, triceps extensions, and quadriceps raises. "Let me show you a new way to work your triceps muscles," says the trainer. Seated, she uses both arms to lift one weight straight up from behind her head, defining the lift as a triceps push-down. All join in. "Remember to breathe, and we'll just do four repetitions of this new one. If your weight seems too heavy for this particular lift, it's okay to go down a pound." The class ends with a collective sigh of relief.

Making a long-term commitment to exercise is a vital component of your success. "You get to a certain fitness level then go two weeks without exercise, and your body is already debilitating back to what it was," says Price. "Two months without exercise and you're back to where you started or even more debilitated."

You may have some worries and fears as you begin pulmonary exercise. The thought of using exercise equipment when you're accustomed to being short of breath with little to no activity may bring some anxious moments, but when you learn that the program is gentle and that with new postures and methods of breathing you can actually use the equipment with success, your

WEEK ONE OF PULMONARY EXERCISE
WHAT TO EXPECT

Your blood pressure, weight, and oxygen saturations will be checked. You will be introduced to aerobic equipment and how to use the rate of perceived exertion (RPE) chart to assign a physical value on your workout. You will use rate of perceived dyspnea (RPD) chart to evaluate your breathing. You will begin a stretching routine and weight training with handheld weights. You may have a relaxation session.

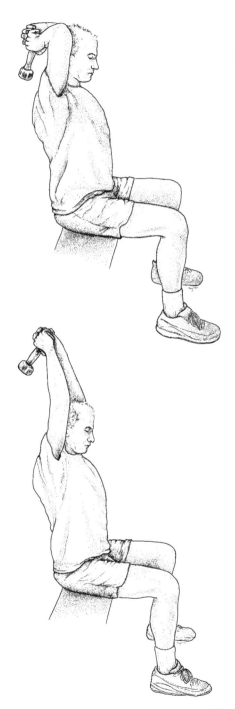

Triceps Push-Down

stress level will decrease. "Patients begin to trust themselves and us and slowly see things changing," says Riddle. "As they are able to get stronger and do more, they're really quite amazed at what they are capable of. They learn to push their own limits. For a lot of people, being out of breath means being out of control. This is all about learning techniques so that they can get control again."

While Bill pushed himself a bit too much and was tired after his first day of Phase II exercise, he remembers finishing his first pulmonary exercise week in high spirits. "I was more confident that I could do the exercise and would eventually gain strength." Now Bill works out three days a week in his wellness maintenance class. "It has been and continues to be a very satisfactory experience," he says. "I think it's what's keeping me alive and moving. Amazingly enough, I look forward to the class."

9

WELLNESS MAINTENANCE EXERCISE

THE PINK HUE of first light streaks across a pale sky. Sounds as familiar as the shuffle of morning slippers permeate the dawn: a barking dog, the insistent mew of a hungry cat, meadowlarks, sirens. The day begins. But this is no ordinary Monday. Challenges have been met, hurdles jumped, goals realized, and significant personal growth achieved. Having completed Phase II wellness education is akin to a life-skills degree. Finishing Phase II wellness exercise is your New York marathon. Today is a day to delight in fulfillment and honor success. You've taken control of your illness and have gained power through knowledge and applied effort. You're on track with diet, you have established a workable routine, and you have greatly improved your level of fitness by adhering to a personal exercise program. Revel in your achievements. Your milestones deserve attention, and so does your future.

Physical conditioning starts to ebb after one week of not working out. After two weeks, the decline back to your old state is well underway. In order to maintain your current fitness status and move ahead, you must continue to exercise. With a diagnosis of heart disease, diabetes, or COPD, exercise in an ongoing, safe environment is the desired situation. In line with the three phase hospital-affiliated wellness program model, Phase III maintenance is a secure, progressive fitness plan—and so much more. There is a talent to combining subtle attention with acute awareness. A well-rounded wellness maintenance team demonstrates this skill.

You are prepared for exercise independence, but the nature of your illness requires diligence. While supporting autonomy, the staff pays close attention to nuance. If someone is working at a slower pace than usual, it will be noticed. A normally vivacious exerciser shifting from exuberance to melancholy will be checked. Questions will be asked if a person looks drawn and pale. And then there's that vexing feeling about a class member that moves the nurse or trainer to exploration beyond casual query. You can't put a name on it, but something's just not right. "This perception is called the thinking gut," says Dr. Smith-Poling. "You have the same neurotransmitters in your gut that are in your brain. So everyone really does have a thinking gut, and until you can resolve whatever the unnamed issue is, it is wise, particularly in a wellness gym setting, to go on it. It has saved lives."

Telemetry is not used in maintenance, but blood pressures are checked weekly (more often in some instances), pulses are taken, and use of rate of perceived exertion (RPE) chart is continued. Diabetics run their own blood glucose tests, but a staff member will consult with them about the numbers, particularly those who are on insulin, or who have a tendency to fluctuate or drop glucose considerably with activity. COPD clients are encouraged to monitor their own oxygen saturation levels before, during, and after exercise, but a trainer or nurse will be close at hand to address any readings below ninety. Patient evaluations will be conducted to keep the staff updated on medications and personal information changes, and to chart present and future goals.

A segue into Phase III maintenance is painless. Whether you are working with the same Phase II staff members or new nurses and trainers, you will start maintenance with the exercise program you were doing at the end of Phase II. If the staff *is* different, there's no cause for distress. You won't be a stranger. When you move into maintenance, an in-depth report goes with you. This will include your medical history, current conditions and medications, personal workout program, physical progress through Phase II exercise, and any issues pertinent to your health and well-being while in maintenance. In conjunction with your current exercise regime, the nurses and trainers will know what the Phase II staff has recommended for your continued fitness advancement, and communication will remain open.

Hours of operation for maintenance vary from program to program. Some run all day, five days a week. Others have morning or afternoon sessions only. There can be structured, assigned classes that last for an hour each, or a daily drop-in schedule. Along with an aerobic workout and training with hand weights, over the course of each week the curriculum can include stretching and relaxation. The number of days per week that you attend will depend on your goals, energy level, physician recommendations, and your availability, as well as the availability of the program. Three days a week is customary, but some people are comfortable with two and others prefer five. Classes are ongoing. You can stay in maintenance indefinitely. For structured classes, your placement depends on the number of people already in the various time slots and your schedule. In some formats, clients are encouraged to record their own activity on an exercise log. Doing so heightens awareness of personal improvements and can add to independence. Other facilities may record all client activity on a computer. There is a nominal fee for maintenance. Like you, your new exercise classmates will all be in the process of strengthening and rebuilding.

You are a different person. Smarter, healthier, and stronger than that first day of Phase II exercise, you enter the maintenance program with a well-earned confidence. You know your workout, the equipment is familiar, and the setting is warm and friendly. While you may not have developed a love for scheduled exercise, or you may still harbor fond memories of the old athletic days of strenuous workouts, those concepts remain on the periphery. What is important today is that your illness is under control, and you are feeling better than you have felt in quite some time. In the early bloom of these healthful facts, commitment to continued fitness is easy. Now comes a crucial time in your new life of regular, reasonable training. This is where the rubber meets the road. You know from your Phase II classes that optimal health and functional independence require a habit of lifelong exercise, but keeping the momentum going and managing mental and physical setbacks are heavy responsibilities. Wellness maintenance is your partner in progress. As a participant in a wellness maintenance program, you become a member of a supportive, uplifting community that shares your highs and lows, respects your hard work, and reinforces your goals and decisions.

Chuck joined wellness exercise after bypass surgery. Six years later, he continues to work out in a maintenance class and says it has helped him establish and maintain a routine of consistent aerobic exercise and improve physical fitness. "I realize as I get older the absolute value of daily exercise in my overall well-being, not only physically but mentally and emotionally." He likes the wellness staff, too. "Having trained supervision is important and valuable. It helps keep me focused on some basics, like doing things properly and safely," Chuck says. He also finds that being a part of the wellness community has benefits beyond fitness. "The social contact with others in the class has added a number of valued new friends to my circle and also a certain obligation to others in the class to reinforce them in their pursuit of well-being."

Decide to get in the habit of showing up for exercise. "We are all ruled by our habits. Whether your habits and their effects are positive or negative depends on your choices. You can choose not to allow your mind to be dominated by negative thoughts. You can make a conscious decision to replace negative ideas and impulses with positive ones whenever they occur. Positive habits will automatically influence your mind to be more alert, your imagination to be more active, your enthusiasm to grow, and your willpower to increase," write Napoleon Hill and Michael J. Ritt, Jr. in Napoleon Hill's *Keys to Positive Thinking*. Once a positive exercise mindset is established, choosing healthy behaviors becomes the focus. With a decision to attend your classes in place, you'll go on the days you'd rather stay home, and even if your workout is less exertive than usual, you'll feel better for the going. Your body will tingle with life, your mind will be alert with the stimulation of conversation, and your spirits will be high in the realization of the decision. Of course, you should stay home if you are genuinely sick, but if you're just feeling droopy and out of sorts, showing up for class can have an energizing effect. "I was never into exercise until I started the wellness program," says eighty-two-year-old

Jean. "Now I enjoy the class so much, and I'm into people so I enjoy the social part. Plus, my doctor says the state of my health is very good, and the exercise probably has a lot to do with it."

After his Phase II cardiac rehabilitation, personal trainer Frank Gentle spent ten years in a variety of different wellness exercise maintenance programs. At the time he became a trainer in 2003, he was working out four to five days a week. "I can't see myself stopping," he says. "The results I get from my doctors are phenomenal. Certainly I'm on all kinds of medications, but the combined results are very positive, so why stop and slide backwards physically, emotionally, and mentally?" As is often the case, the sense of community in wellness exercise is a big draw for Gentle. "The environment is very supportive. It's not a group-hug type of thing, but if a person doesn't show up there are concerns. Is so-and-so okay?" As mentioned earlier in chapter four, the actual act of exercising can become an aside to the group dynamic. "You can walk on a treadmill and get into some pretty good discussions for fifteen or twenty minutes," says Gentle. "You talk to someone you enjoy and get to exercise, and you don't notice you're exercising." Gentle feels lucky to have survived a heart attack and to have wended his way through some more years of his life to become a wellness personal trainer. "This works for me probably better than when I made a whole lot more money. I'm dealing with my peers and I'm involved in doing something I really enjoy." And how does he motivate his wellness clients? "You have to feel that you have something to offer. You have to be sincere and show you can do it, and you do that by proving yourself. Clients relate well to knowing my health background. I'm obviously one of them. I've been through serious problems and survived."

IT'S MONDAY MORNING maintenance. In this particular facility, the maintenance program is called Exercise for Health. There are six structured one-hour classes held each weekday. The gym ambience is warm and friendly. Hardy green plants adorn desks, countertops, and corners. Stretching charts, postings for upcoming forums, health articles, and cartoons abound. Red, green, purple, and pink hand weights line one wall and resistance bands dangle from another. A mountain of yellow and blue exercise balls balances behind a workout bench. On the other side of the room, rays of warm sunshine stream in through a wall of windows illuminating the array of treadmills, upright bicycles, recumbent bikes, a rower, hand cycle and elliptical mechanism, and an abdominal crunch machine. Outside, the turquoise bay glistens in the blaze of a summer morning.

The first class members to arrive bustle through the doors engrossed in animated conversation that likely began in the elevator. The banter centers on a plethora of grandkid photos. "Look how cute he is here. He's definitely the best looking baby," says one granddad. "Wait a minute," a gal pipes up. "Just take a look at these pictures of our twins." Other members of the group aren't far behind. One woman brings a bouquet from her garden—red and white rhododendrons. Another helps Sam, an elderly gentleman, with his walker. A retired doctor who attends the class brings medical articles on cardiac diet and fitness for the trainer to read and post. The last two exercisers straggle in—engrossed in a music discussion. One has a portable oxygen tank slung over his shoulder. He plays the saxophone in a local jazz band.

Folks get checked in: blood pressures for everyone, blood glucose numbers for the diabetics, oxygen saturations for pulmonary clients. Some take their own pulses, the trainer assists others. "I get to hold a lot of hands when I take pulses in my groups," says Gentle. "People find it comforting. One of the most important things seems to be human contact." Sam's pulse is elevated and irregular today, and he's a little short of breath. The nurse is called into the gym to evaluate him further. Exercise logs are pulled, and most of the class takes over recording their own vitals and workout stats.

Treadmills, bicycles, and recumbent bikes whir. The topics of conversation run from a sugar-free applesauce muffin recipe to cars and the latest movies playing downtown. The room hums with rhythm. The trainer circulates and chats with everyone individually. The banter is light, but questions are worked into the exchange. "How's that knee feeling today? Tell me what's going on with your new diet. You're not walking as fast as usual, what's up?" On the other side of the room, the nurse has run a cardiogram strip on Sam and is calling his doctor.

Forty-five minutes into the session, the class gravitates to the weight training area of the gym. Everyone independently begins stretching - standing lunges, toe raises, the quadriceps and calf stretch, arm circles, and raised arm and shoulder. One of the diabetes clients stops to have some juice that he brought from home. Sam's daughter-in-law arrives to take him to the doctor. He gets a rousing "good luck" from classmates.

WELLNESS MAINTENANCE

Ongoing and safe, with an enjoyable ambience, wellness maintenance supports your independence and continued commitment to optimal health.

Before long, each person is wielding a set of hand weights. "What should we talk about while we use these bloody things?" asks one of the men. "Let's talk about our fearless leader. She's always a good target," jokes another. The trainer has everyone stand up. "Well, if you're going to talk about me, it's going to be while doing your lifts standing and adding at least six repetitions to each one," she threatens, with a sly grin. The class quiets down, mumbling and slinking back into chairs. They decide to talk about the city councilman who has the town in a buzz. It seems his faux pas involves making a questionable public comment about a questionable public figure. Eight biceps curls, triceps extensions, upright rows, military presses, triceps push-downs, shoulder shrugs, and side bends later, the rowdy discussion shows no sign of ending. "Don't put your weights away yet," the trainer says. "Since you're all so full of life, let's do two more lifts." Without skipping a beat in the hot debate, they balance the weights on their legs and execute four quadriceps raises and four toe raises, first right and then left.

Resting pulses, blood glucose numbers, and oxygen saturations are appropriately checked. Exercise logs are completed with workout information and final vitals, and the assembly gravitates to the elevator with the city councilman's indiscretion the exit topic.

In keeping with the concept of lifetime fitness, it is important to mention maintenance and moving. After months, or years, of participating in your wellness maintenance exercise program, you are making plans to relocate. It may be a job transfer to a different state, retirement, getting closer to or farther away from family, or joining the migration to warmer climates. In the flurry of activity, be sure to include the task of getting established in a new wellness exercise class. This will require a medical referral from your new healthcare provider. To assist in the transition, you, or your current physician, should request copies of at least the last several months of your wellness exercise logs. This information can then be included in your medical records that are transferred to your new physician. Once your new doctor has checked your current health status and reviewed your records, the exercise history will help him/her in the referral process.

Mastering a chronic illness, completing Phase II wellness, and becoming a member of maintenance exercise are undertakings to savor. You have climbed mountains. What an incredible journey. Plodding through the surreal first days of diagnosis, disbelief, and dismay, you have found your way. Your willingness to work toward a state of improved health is a personal gift and a public example. Your determination is to be congratulated, admired, and respected. "Adopting an exercise mindset is part of changing your whole orientation," says Dr. David Whitney. "Once it is habit, it won't seem like climbing mountains, it will just become part of your life."

> *"In the last analysis, our only freedom is the freedom to discipline ourselves." —Bernard Baruch*

10

ADDING TO THE LIFE OF FITNESS

SO, YOU'RE IN FOR the long haul. You have increased your exercise tolerance and strengthened all of your muscles. You've gained a wealth of knowledge regarding your chronic illness and have made some new friends along the way. In orchestrating a lifestyle conducive to optimal health, you have learned the importance of keeping on track and sticking to training, but let's take a realistic look at committing to a lifetime of exercise. While the habit of fitness is firmly in place, every now and then the drill gets boring. You try to spice things up by using different machines or buying a new pair of workout shoes, but BORING hammers at your resolve. Your wellness team may have the cure. Many wellness departments offer such extended services as yoga, therapeutic massage, balance classes, and even advanced weight training that, in conjunction with your regular exercise program, will bolster your commitment, rev up enthusiasm, promote continued good health, and give your mind and body a well-deserved gift.

A yoga class is an ideal addition to a goal of physical health and inner harmony. Yoga means union—integration. The practice of yoga brings together the mental, emotional, spiritual, and physical body. "When I teach yoga, the kind of experience I'm looking for is one where the physical body is engaged and is experiencing and growing toward the body's limit or comfort range," says instructor Gary Lemons. "It may look nothing like a picture you've seen, and it may be nothing like what the person next to you is doing, but the inner experience is that you're fully present in the moment and not hurting yourself. Then the mental and emotional body comes along and acts in harmony with the physical body."

Yoga is diverse in its application from gentle to aerobic, and the practice can complement other forms of therapy and exercise. If you're dealing with pulmonary disease, there are various yoga breathing techniques that settle and quiet the mind which, in turn, will quiet the heart and lower blood pressure. Depending on your stage of recovery, you can just do the breathing practice and no other physical yoga. "The breathing is very powerful because the breath keeps us alive," says Lemons. "If you get into the gentle rhythm and let the wave of the breath come through you, the whole organic being will become peaceful. Breathing is a constant in and out that is a way of understanding our own preciousness and relevance to the universe."

> ## YOGA
>
> Yoga complements therapies and exercises for heart disease, diabetes, and COPD with slow to vigorous standing poses, positions to enhance circulation, and breathing techniques. The exercise of yoga breathing can support the concept of daily aerobic activity.

In addition to the breathing techniques, which are also critical components of yoga for cardiac and diabetes patients, standing yoga poses are great for you if your health issue is heart disease. The poses can be done very slowly or vigorously to accommodate your stage of recovery. During the movements, you allow the breath to be the engine by which the physical body responds. "If the breath is allowed to drive the body, the body will be much safer than if the mind does," says Lemons. "The mind has a tendency to judge and have expectations that are unrealistic."

Because circulation is an issue for you if you have diabetes, elevation of the feet coupled with very slow yoga movements and stretches is a good way to start. Working within the comfort limits of your disease, over time your stretches will become deeper and your body will open more to the movements.

The practice of yoga doesn't necessarily require you to be physical, you can choose to just be present in the moment, sit for twenty minutes, and breathe. That simplicity can be the catalyst that rids you of your exercise doldrums. Just sitting and doing proper yoga breathing frees you from the requirement of a physical conclusion. "By being liberated from the expectation of having to do something physical every day, you end up feeling like doing it," says Lemons. "The feeling of self-empowerment creates a willingness to be disciplined."

Therapeutic massage by a trained therapist is another modality that can reinforce your wellness commitment and help to manage and possibly improve your health status.

Massage covers a number of techniques of hands-on therapy or body work. Some approaches that are beneficial to people with chronic illness include polarity therapy, zero balancing, strain/counter strain, craniosacral, myofascial release, visceral massage, trigger point therapy, neuromuscular therapy, acupressure, polarity therapy, energy work, Feldenkrais, and reflexology. "Many of these techniques are not circulatory; that is, they do not move blood and lymph and are, therefore, not apt to

MASSAGE

The physical benefits of massage include:
1. Relaxed muscles, elimination of spasms, a boost to energy, softening of connective tissue, an increase in range of motion by freeing up the joints
2. Promotion of circulation that improves the flow of nutrients, oxygen, hormones, antibodies, and water to the cells and carries away waste products
3. Decrease in pain
4. Release of "feel good" hormones
5. Increase in immune system functioning

The mental and emotional benefits of massage include:
1. Decreased depression
2. Decreased anxiety
3. Increased relaxation
4. Increased mental clarity
5. Increased self-esteem

overload the system of a person with a severe illness," says Jan Burr, a licensed massage practitioner who works with wellness clients. A chronically ill person must not be over-treated. "In order to provide the most beneficial treatment, the massage practitioner working with a chronically ill person needs to be aware of the medications the person is taking and must understand the chronic illness patterns and the affects of the medications involved," says Burr. "With regular massage, a person may not improve physically yet they may have a better quality of life, experience less tension and stress and, therefore, be better able to cope with the illness. You want the client to achieve the highest quality of life possible."

Anxiety produces muscle tension. Tight muscles cause pain, and pain leads to more anxiety. Therapeutic, nurturing touch can break the cycle. "Many people I meet in my practice complain they don't know how to relax. They hold their shoulders up to their ears, clench their jaw, squint their eyes, and brace themselves in a chair," says Burr. "Touch to these areas of tension gives sensory feedback to the brain. Over time a person can learn to release the tension and eventually learn to notice on their own when they are carrying tension and let it go. Regular massage, thus, can break up physical and mental holding patterns; it is a whole body experience."

Adding massage therapy to your wellness exercise regime can help with the recovery time of sore muscles and prevent overuse injuries that, in turn, enables you to avoid any interruption in exercise routine. "By receiving massage, you learn to be kind to your body, pace, listen to pain, and modify exercises daily to prevent fatigue and injury," adds Burr. "Massage and exercise programs are ways of increasing a person's hardiness."

In dealing with diabetes, COPD, and heart disease, Burr offers these guidelines for safe, effective massage.

For the diabetic with healthy, resilient tissue, a moderate Swedish massage could be appropriate. Those with less healthy tissue would benefit from non-circulatory techniques. Massage must be avoided at the site of the last insulin injection. Also, the therapist must be aware of diminished sensation due to peripheral neuropathy so as not to over-treat or injure tissues.

In the early stages of COPD, a circulatory massage may be appropriate if tissues are healthy. Back, neck, and chest massage may be most helpful. Gentle myofascial release (MFR) to these areas, as well as release of the rib cage and diaphragm can help. For more advanced cases in which there's trouble breathing, more calming techniques may reduce anxiety and fatigue. Passive joint movements of the head and shoulders can release tension. As COPD patients are often not comfortable lying down, massage in a semi-reclining or seated position would be best. No scented oils or fragrances would be used.

While traditional Swedish circulatory massage may overload the system of someone with heart problems, many cardiac patients participating in a regular exercise program are healthier than they were before, making circulatory massage appropriate. One index of ability to withstand circulation massage is the level of doctor-approved activity. Gentle myofascial release or scar tissue release if a person has had heart surgery may decrease the tight feeling in the chest and improve breathing. Gentle touching of the scarring may release emotions that could reduce anxiety and fear. Also, trigger point therapy can help release painful areas in specific muscles. Massage must be avoided where any clotting or plaques have formed. Clients taking blood thinners may be at risk for bruising, making lighter pressure during massage a necessity.

The massage practitioner working with diabetes, cardiac, and COPD clients must obtain an informed consent from the physician and must also stay updated on client condition in order to make necessary adjustments to the type of massage given. "Every chronically ill person can benefit from appropriate nurturing, listening, and skilled touch," Burr says. "The right technique can be found for each individual. With decreased pain and anxiety levels, one is more likely to continue with an exercise program. Massage combined with exercise may reduce the impact of disease on one's life."

Retired physical therapist Barbara Paschal has developed a balance aerobic program that is an ideal addition to wellness exercise. A balance class can bring variety to your fitness routine, encourage new interest in personal health goals, and add an element of confidence to your workout. In her book *Balance Aerobics*, Paschal writes, "Balance is now the focus of a great deal of research primarily focusing on prevention of frequent falls. The research also shows that balance can be improved! How much each person can improve is quite individual. And it will be well worth your efforts. And it can be fun! Plus, along the way you will also improve your strength, flexibility, endurance and coordination."

> ## BALANCE CLASS
>
> You will gain balance and confidence. You will develop better movement practices, have less fear of falling, and improve flexibility and coordination.

Weakness and poor range of motion can occur after surgery and with chronic illness. Being physically off balance is common. "Fear of falling is one of the biggest reasons for balance deficit," says Paschal. "People need more exercise and more practice in moving in a balanced fashion. They're afraid, therefore balance strategies become inappropriate, but understandable." Balance can be relearned. "When you have better movement practices, you won't be afraid of falling." Reaching, stepping, walking with proper form, the balance class movements mimic real life set to music.

The balance aerobics class consists of a thirty minute lecture on balance, walking, posture, how to prevent pain and injury, and strengthening various areas of the body. Fifty minutes of the class are devoted to a moderate, low-impact aerobic set of exercises that focus on balance. Each session includes a warm-up and cool down employing the same aerobic movements as in the workout, but in slower motion. "There's constant repetition, and research has found that repetition improves balance. There must be a great deal of practice. It's much like learning to play the piano, if you were to go for lessons for the first time you'd be asked to practice," says Paschal. "Where the mind and the body merge, which is very much balance, one must practice. Then your brain begins to lay down the memory of the correct movements. Balance does diminish somewhat with age, but what they have found is that we are speeding up that diminishment of balance not with age, but with what we do with age."

A balance class is a good motivator for continuing wellness fitness. Renewed confidence not only increases comfort levels when doing daily chores, but also when engaging in exercise. With better balance, you will move about the gym more confidently and get on and off equipment in a steadier motion. Also, the class reinforces the fun of fitness. "When you move with a bunch of people in a room there's a bonding, and we laugh," says Paschal. "I encourage laughter. It's good for every part of you. My life as a physical therapist has allowed me the privilege of helping others see that they can improve despite severe injuries, surgeries, birth defects, and diseases. I am absolutely convinced that our bodies and especially our brains are amazing, and that the human spirit is capable of tremendous things!"

If you have health factors that prohibit the physical movement of upright balance training, a modified approach to tai chi may be a way for you to add energy and diversity to your fitness program.

Tai chi, a Chinese term, translates to universal harmony. It is represented by the yin/yang symbol (also known as the tai chi circle) that indicates opposing yet interactive and complementary aspects of the natural world. "Health and optimal function are based on the harmony of yin and yang, and this balanced state can be called tai chi," says tai chi chuan instructor Andrew G. Holmes. "The Chinese view is that the cosmos, including human existence, is an evolutionary process of constant cyclical change. With these forces always in motion together, opportunities exist for recovering and sustaining balance. The natural result of this process is greater health and growth."

The term tai chi is a shortened phrase for tai chi chuan (TCC), a potent martial art that is the physical practice of expressing yin and yang energy through meditative movements used as a system of daily exercise. "Practitioners of TCC are doing a comprehensive form of chi kung (energy work) in which they gain body awareness through repetitive movements and understanding of the interaction between yin and yang," says Holmes. "Regular practice creates an atmosphere in the body that is favorable to self-healing, through the development of internal energy. Automatic progress results from continued practice and proper training." Along with the physical rewards, tai chi chuan can add a mental and emotional component. "Continued practice helps students understand changes within the body relative to the outside world," says Holmes. "There are benefits related to stress reduction, as TCC is an excellent relaxation technique, in addition to the more typical benefits gained from regular weight bearing exercise and aerobic conditioning."

Holmes, who has been interested in health and personal development for more than twenty years, teaches five tai chi classes each week. One of his classes is specifically designed for students with chronic conditions that prohibit standing for long periods of time. "This class doesn't have the martial training component, so it is more appropriately labeled as chi kung, rather than tai chi chuan," Holmes says. "Students still seem to improve balance and get some of the other benefits from regular TCC, but curriculum is limited to upper body movement, with the objective of energy circulation without so much focus on manifesting power and applying it physically in self-defense. Students can still reap some of the benefits of TCC movement without really getting into the deeper martial levels or meditative aspect of more intense training."

The one-hour long program, suitable for stroke survivors, folks with Parkinson's disease and multiple sclerosis, as well as those with diabetes, heart disease, and COPD, allows students to remain seated throughout the class. The exercises are simple and relaxing.

"The benefits come from waist-oriented movements, which are at the core of all authentic styles of TCC," Holmes says. "With feet firmly planted flat on the ground, and sitting squarely, students turn ribs left and right throughout most postures. This activates the waist area. These movements are good because the internal organs are energized by increased circulation and slow breathing. The postures involve balanced arm movements generated from the waist turns, and there is also a component of spinal flexion. Using the back like this, to assist the upper body in opening and closing, results in the most dynamic expression of the postures, and maximizes the physical changes from yin and yang." According to Holmes, this becomes like a gentle form of aerobic exercise for the vital organs. "As a result of this kind of nourishment, chemical processes happen more efficiently," he adds. "With consistent practice, digestion is also improved, and blood pressure reduced. Students also report being more at ease during flare-ups of their symptoms, and are able to maintain a more focused mind state."

For you, as a participant in a hospital-affiliated aerobic and weight training exercise program, the addition of seated tai chi can add a new dimension to wellness. Holmes feels that TCC and chi kung forms, in general, have great application as cross training or supplemental conditioning when taught along with more conventional exercise. The movements are low-impact, and, due to the increased body awareness that students develop, are beneficial as forms of physical therapy, because participants get into a more relaxed state-of-mind that can contribute to healing. "The psychological benefits are often overlooked, as people typically grasp for physical solutions," says Holmes. "Students who practice regularly learn deeper lessons through this kind of simple exercise and breathing than just how to perform physical movements. Certain autogenic phenomena develop through repetitive movements. In addition to the physical side and social interaction, students seem to get an imprint in the consciousness of what it feels like to relax in the body and the mind. This is empowering, and provides internal support and motivation to face other challenges in life."

When considering a tai chi class, it is important to study with someone who continues to develop and improve their own skills and understanding, advises Holmes. "I recommend avoiding instructors who are more focused on enrollment than quality of

TAI CHI

Tai chi is a shortened phrase for tai chi chuan (TCC), a potent martial art. Seated tai chi is a modified version that offers you a good cross training activity. It can help your circulation, increase your body awareness, and promote a relaxed state of mind.

instruction and individual growth." Holmes continues to study under Master Alex Dong of New York. "I would have nothing to offer if it wasn't for the teachers who taught me previously and continue to train me today."

Occasionally the "boring" aspect of a long-term wellness maintenance exercise routine can develop as a direct result of physical improvement. You may be a person who is able to make tremendous strides in your level of fitness. Each six-month evaluation is better than the last, and an increase in your aerobic workout is regularly approved. Thoughts of

ADVANCED WEIGHT TRAINING

Your benefits will be an increase in conditioning, a broader personal fitness information base, and autonomy without risk.

dropping out and joining a gym or exercising on your own arise. You think you'd like to have the freedom to work hard without intervention, but you know you would lose the guidance that a hands-on staff affords, as well as the comfort that comes with the reassuring tone of wellness. "Sometimes I feel I've outgrown this place, but I know someone will always be here to help me just in case something goes wrong," says one exerciser of long standing. There is a solution. Advanced weight training classes for appropriate clients can be part of the maintenance program. Wellness Director Schmidt advises that those best qualified for an advanced supervised class are persons with the least amount of damage from a heart attack, those who had a higher level of physical functioning before their "event," and those whose pulmonary function will support it. From her observations of an advanced class, Schmidt says, "It provided more variety, challenge, and level of fitness for those whose physical conditioning allowed. People who took it really liked it. It gave them the tools to work independently."

Certified personal trainer and wellness exercise technician Barbara Vane has taught an advanced weight training class to her physically able people who wanted to add to the life of their fitness with a more strenuous program. "There seemed to be some interest from a few clients, so I thought I'd give it a chance." The class was held once a week for one month. "I determined the intensity of the workout based on each client's exercise history, their age and general condition, and by their ability at the lightest weights to have good form and be able to complete a set of repetitions without failure," says Vane. "Increases were made slowly, according to the ability of each client to maintain good form as weight loads were increased." As they progressed, they were invited to incorporate the new routine into their regular wellness maintenance workout by reducing aerobic activity and using the time to do their accelerated weightlifting in the established class, but on their own. "I went from excited to intimidated back to excited," says Henry. "I really wanted to advance my weight training, but wasn't sure I could handle the class. When I saw my improvements at the end of the month, I was really pleased." The end results for someone wanting more of a weight training challenge, while remaining in the secure setting of the wellness gym, are an increase in conditioning, a broader personal fitness information base, and autonomy without risk.

> ## SUPPORT GROUPS
>
> You will enjoy discussions, speakers, and added education through a positive platform of continued growth and advancement in the governing of your chronic illness.

If your wellness maintenance program does not offer an advanced class and you feel you are stagnating at you current level of exercise, make the suggestion before you bolt. It may be a way to have the best of both worlds.

Many wellness programs have support groups for their clients. Some may be called "Better Breathers," "Diabetes Diatribe," "Heart Savers." Once-a-month meetings may include group discussions and questions, as well as guest speakers who have new medical information or share ideas and personal experiences. Getting together with others who are dealing with similar health issues improves moral, adds to education, and creates a positive platform for continued growth and advancement in the governing of chronic illness. If you are in a program that does not have a support group for your needs, play an active role in getting one started. Share your idea with the staff. They may be willing to scout up a qualified facilitator to organize and oversee the meetings.

The hospital affiliated wellness program is a voyage to optimal fitness and health for cardiac, diabetes, and COPD clients. Providing a safe, caring, knowledgeable environment, the wellness program educates, supports, and motivates participants to manage their illness, reach attainable goals, and foster a brighter future. It is a program dedicated to you, but keeping the momentum going is an individual responsibility. You, too, must be dedicated. Use the program thoroughly and wisely. Explore everything it has to offer and become an active participant in upholding your health. Find your niche, forge new paths, and celebrate your accomplishments. Your wellness team is rooting for you. Stay in the game and make every day a winner. Go for the wellness gold of maximum fitness with minimum risk.

11

SHARING THE ROAD TO WELLNESS

IT WAS A FRESH FALL New England morning in 1984. A yellow sun glistened on the thick red and gold landscape of the valley. The crisp autumn breeze drifted through an open window with the scent of enkindled oak from toasty fireplaces and wood stoves. I was sitting with two neighbors in the quiet of a Connecticut kitchen sipping coffee and nibbling toasted bagels. In the middle of the conversation about children and our precarious sanity, one of the women burst into tears and on to a completely different subject.

"I just have to tell someone or I'll explode," she said. "I went to a health fair last month and found out my blood pressure is sky high and so is my cholesterol. My blood glucose is out of whack, and I'm overweight. They said I am a prime candidate for a heart attack. I'm scared to death."

My other neighbor reached across the table, took the woman's two hands in hers, and gave them a tight, loving squeeze.

"You know, my blood pressure and cholesterol used to be pretty high," she said. "I was overweight, too. After I fretted about those facts, I got into a good diet and exercise routine, and I got better."

Like the slow drawing of a curtain on a clear, new day, the tension lifted from my frightened neighbor's body. She exhaled with a loud whoosh, her tight shoulders dropped, and her taut face muscles relaxed into a smile.

"I can't believe it," she gushed. "You're so healthy and fit. I just thought you were one of those lucky people without problems. You've made me feel so much better, like I'm not doomed, like I can do something, too."

In the bucolic setting of a country kitchen, over morning coffee and easy communion, I was witness to a powerful moment. An uncertain path became less rocky, because one person divulged a piece of her soul and tempered the fright in another person's mind. My neighbor's openness made it apparent that everyone has the opportunity to assist and strengthen others by the simple act of sharing. It is a cost-free contribution that enriches the community. For people who find themselves suddenly dealing with chronic illness, the shared experience is a gift.

Holly Short

Heart disease is the number-one killer of women in the United States. It claims more lives each year than all types of cancer combined. Although women are becoming more health savvy in regard to heart disease, the diagnosis can still pack a wallop. Wellness exercise client Holly Short didn't expect to be sidelined by a heart attack at the age of fifty-six. I chatted with her recently about her event.

cm: Tell me about the day you had your heart attack, Holly.
hs: I had my heart attack on May 31, 1997. It was just a normal day. The weather was sunny and warm - a perfect day for working in the yard. I only came in for lunch. About 5 p.m., I started getting a headache. This didn't bother me as I am prone to them, but the headache got stronger, so I took a couple of aspirin and decided to lie down. The headache kept getting worse, and then I started sweating. I began to worry that I was having a stroke. Finally, I called 911. For me, that was a difficult phone call to make. I had no symptoms of a heart attack, and I didn't want to call an ambulance and have it turn out that all I had was a migraine. I was told later that if I had waited five more minutes it would have been too late.

cm: Did you expect this would ever happen to you?
hs: I never thought it would be me. What stupidity! My dad had heart problems, my younger brother had had two heart attacks, and

my mom died of a heart attack, but I didn't think of it for me. I was on medication for high blood pressure, and as long as I took it, my numbers were good. Looking back, I think my doctor should have been more aware—given my history. I don't remember having my lipids checked or any serious talks about weight, exercise, or my smoking.

cm: A high percentage of women don't survive a cardiac event. How do you feel about being a heart attack survivor?

hs: Very lucky. Personally, I think one of the reasons women don't survive is that we don't always have the standard symptoms. I had no chest pressure or pain down my arm. Women need to become more aware of the full range of symptoms that can mean the onset of an attack.

cm: What motivates you to share your heart experience with others?

hs: Any knowledge that I have that can help save a heart attack victim from death is more than enough reason to share my experience.

cm: What were your exercise habits before your heart attack?

hs: None, zilch, nada. Work took all I had. The only exercise I got was walking my dog, Honey, and that wasn't more than a block.

cm: How soon after your heart attack did you get involved in a wellness program?

hs: While I was still in the hospital, one of the medical people gave me the name of a wellness person she knew. When I got back home and felt strong enough (I think it was a couple of months) I called her up, and the rest is history. She was a very easy person to talk to during a difficult time. As you know, when you enter cardiac rehab it isn't just exercise. They get you every which way but loose, which is good. There is nutrition, mental health, stress discussion, medications, etc. All bases are covered.

cm: Why did you decide to commit to wellness exercise?

hs: I had finally realized that if I wanted to continue to live, I had better get on the ball. Part of that was exercise. I also liked the idea, since I had just had a heart attack, that I would be monitored. There would be people in wellness who would know what to look for and keep tabs on me. That was important then, and it still is now.

cm: How did you feel on those first days in the wellness gym? Any intimidation?

hs: Yes, the first days in the wellness gym were a bit intimidating, but the staff soon made me feel at home. All of the equipment was explained, how to operate, etc. Before long, I felt like a pro.

cm: Tell me about your overall wellness exercise experience.

hs: I have nothing but good things to say about wellness exercise. With the machines, weights, and once-a-week meditation, it's a great combination of physical and mental. After all, machines are great, but the mind needs a workout too, needs to keep a positive attitude. The program is a good overall package.

cm: Since your move to Arizona, are you continuing to exercise in a wellness program?

hs: Yes, I am continuing in a wellness program here in Arizona.

cm: So, how are you doing, seven years after your heart attack? How was your last cardiology exam?

hs: My last tests were great. My new cardiologist said whatever I had been doing, keep it up. Since wellness exercise was what I was doing, I guess I had better keep my nose to the grindstone.

cm: What advice do you have for people with chronic illness who might be skeptical about joining a wellness exercise program?

hs: Do it! Just try it for a month and you will notice a decided difference in your abilities. Everything will flow or move better. Maybe you will lift a bag of groceries without huffing, walk a little farther, or get up from a chair a little easier. Whatever your chronic illness, the program will help make life much easier for you.

cm: Anything else you would like to add about exercise and heart disease, or diabetes, or lung disease?

hs: I guess it all boils down to what you want your quality of life to be. I know someone who had a heart attack and now just sits and knits, reads, and watches TV. Each year, I notice she is moving slower—and talking now about a wheelchair. It's sad, because her husband is still very active, and she loved to garden.

I wonder what she would be like today if she had gone to an exercise program.

Jerry Stein

Our paths are all different, but we can make them easier.
Although he doesn't think he really "deals" with illness, exerciser Jerry Stein shares his story and his views.

cm: Jerry, tell me about your health issues.
js: It's probably easier to say what don't I have. I had a heart attack in 1975. I had aortic iliac bypass surgery in 1982. I also have what I'm told is interstitial lung disease.

cm: Tell me about your heart attack in 1975.
js: Shortly after lunch, I was walking down Fifth Avenue in New York with my business partner. I felt like I had terrible indigestion, and I collapsed on the street. I was taken to a hospital and understand that I was unconscious for about thirty-six hours. The one thing that I really noticed when I became conscious was that I had no fear. I guess some would say that's the essence of denial, or for me a belief in destiny. I sort of had the feeling that what was supposed to be with me was going to be, so it did not impact me, or what I did.

cm: What about your lung disease?
js: As a child, I had pneumonia and bronchitis often, and I've always had lung problems. The Army found spots on my lung when they took a chest x-ray during out-processing. They thought I had TB and didn't want to let me out. My doctor convinced them to let me out. Then maybe seven or ten years later, I was denied life insurance after a chest X-ray. They said I had congestive heart failure, and I said I don't think that's my problem. I thought they were nuts. When I moved to California in 1978, I found a cardiologist who made me go for some lung tests. I was diagnosed with interstitial lung disease, probably from my previous experiences as a kid.

cm: When I approached you to do this interview, you said you didn't really deal with illness. What did you mean by that?
js: When I first learned that I needed aortic bypass surgery, I

couldn't work, I couldn't do anything, I was so uptight about it. I feared the process—the thought of going through the processes of an illness, the tests, etc. I was not as frightened of the bypass procedure as I was of getting there. One reason may be that my father had cancer and went through chemotherapy and it was a very difficult period. I remember his process. I would rather keel over in the street than have to go through the process of an illness. I rarely think of illness itself.

cm: Do you think that's a form of denial?

js: You're calling it denial. I'm not sure I'm calling it denial. It goes along with the way I think my life is and the way I think the world is; that everybody is driven by their higher self and that there is very little control over life. I was in a discussion group once where the leader asked, "What is your purpose in life?" People responded with things like, "do good every day," or "try every day to do something to help humanity." He asked me and I said, "My purpose in life is to be and experience." That's what I believe, and whatever I'm drawn to do, I do, not because I think about it, but because I just go from day to day "being." I've never planned my life. I live moment to moment.

cm: So with the attitude of "being and experiencing," how did you land in wellness exercise?

js: I didn't say to myself that getting into wellness was going to be good for me, so I'm going to spend six years doing it. I just did it with no forethought. I'm sure somebody said, hey, there's a wellness program if you want to join, but my subconscious told me to do it. My subconscious tells me to take these stupid pills. While I must be going to wellness for my health, because why the hell else would I do it, that isn't consciously why I do it. Something inside of me tells me to do it. And you also have to understand that my wife talks every day, she tells me things. I think I don't listen —maybe I do, but I truly believe that it is my soul that tells me to come up with these things, and that I will go through whatever I have to go through. I'm here in this human body to experience for the benefit of my soul, whatever my soul is—a little piece of a higher being, or whatever. I'm here for a purpose, and that is to "be" so that my soul can experience.

cm: What have you gotten out of wellness exercise?
js: I've gotten camaraderie, which helps reduce stress. I suppose if I was not doing it, I wouldn't be able to do some of the things I do, but I haven't compared the two.

cm: Any last comments on health?
js: I look at my health life, and I have a lot of opportunities. If I were to analyze it intellectually, I'm probably about in the middle. I'm less into taking care of myself than many and more into taking care of myself than many, so, through no fault of my consciousness, I've ended up in a middle-of-the road place. I don't give up a lot of what I find enjoyable in life, but I'm not sitting on the couch smoking cigars and having beers.

cm: What motivates you to share your experiences?
js: Because you asked, and because I thought it would be fun. I have no motivation to better the world because of it. If you and your readers are interested in how a very different person deals with these issues - and I don't consider it "dealing" because I don't feel like I'm doing it as a planned something - I somehow seem to fall in the middle, which I'm basically happy about.

cm: Anything else you'd like to add?
js: Would you like my views on politics?

cm: How about just your views on wellness exercise.
js: I like the people.

Frank Norwood

Eighty-nine-year-old diabetes client Frank Norwood has participated in a wellness exercise program for more than nine years.

cm: When were you diagnosed with diabetes?
fn: About ten years ago. I had gone to my urologist for my annual checkup and he thought something was amiss in my blood work, so he told me to see my regular doctor. Sure enough, I had signs of diabetes. So it all started from there.
cm: Was it difficult to accept the diagnosis?
fn: I didn't expect it, but it wasn't too difficult to accept. I've had my shot at life. I turned eight-nine last month. That's a long time

to hang around. My mother was a hundred and four when she died, and two sisters are in their nineties.

cm: Once you were diagnosed, what lifestyle adjustments did you make?
fn: Eating, for one thing, and starting a regular fitness regime. I followed what the doctor told me to do and not to do.

cm: How long after your diagnosis did you get involved in a diabetes education and exercise program?
fn: Almost immediately. My diabetes educator put me in her classes, and then I went into maintenance exercise.

cm: How did you find out about the diabetes educator in your area?
fn: My doctor sent me to her.

cm: When you first started diabetes wellness exercise, did you like it?
fn: I think I tolerated it. It was a change in my priorities and way of living and what I did. I thought, well, I'll hang on to this for a little while—maybe I'll attend, and maybe I won't. And then somebody got it into my head that if I wanted to stick around a little longer, I'd better get into the exercise and stay with it. At my age and with my habits, I have a lot of time if I want to devote it to what I should, so I got into it, and I enjoy it now.

cm: Have you ever thought about giving it up?
fn: Not really, not about quitting. I kind of thought once in a while I'll go and once in a while I won't, but now I attend quite regularly. In the spring, I drop one day a week and go out and play golf. Hopefully, I get enough exercise doing that. In the fall, I go back to three days a week of wellness exercise.

cm: What was your motivation for getting into an exercise program?
fn: My diabetes educator gave me the motivation. "Get into it or you're not going to get well, or even stay steady," she said.

cm: What were your exercise habits before diabetes and wellness exercise?
fn: Really not much of anything other than playing golf, and once

in a while I'd go walking. I'd walk off and on because I was packing on a little extra weight, but if the weather was bad, I wouldn't get out.

cm: What have you gotten out of the wellness exercise program?
fn: I've gotten a lot of knowledge about this diabetes business. I've met some very good people, both instructors and fellow patients. I look forward to going to class. I get there early just to talk. It's pleasant, you learn a lot about each other. The exercise, and the fact that I have a doctor that keeps track of me, helps control my diabetes.

cm: Does your doctor support your involvement in exercise?
fn: Oh yes, yes indeed. He's very adamant about it.

cm: What motivates you to continue?
fn: I guess a fear of getting high blood glucose numbers and not really knowing what will happen if I don't do it. And the camaraderie. You know, it's no longer a chore to go. It's a pleasure to go now. We have a lot of fun.

cm: Does adherence to a regular exercise program help you to get out and play golf and enjoy other activities?
fn: I think so, but I am getting old, you know. I don't have the muscle memory that I had before. I do work in the yard a lot. I'm sure the whole exercise program is the reason I'm able to do what I'm able to do. If I had taken the idea of oh, the hell with it, I'll go if and when I want to, I wouldn't be sitting here talking to you, I don't believe.

cm: Any advice for others with diabetes who are considering wellness exercise?
fn: Yes. Get into it as quick as you can and stay with it.

cm: What inspires you to share your story?
fn: I think anybody who has this malady should take any opportunity to let people know their story. It's worth the time and the effort. The exercise has been very beneficial for me. Otherwise, I'd probably be a couch potato and not talking to you now.
The experiences and attitudes of clients involved in the wellness exercise community are varied and unique, but there is a strong

uniting force. Everyone is working with some sort of health issue. When there is sharing, the load is lightened. Chronic illness doesn't have to be a solo journey.

———⟫●⟪———

12

CONFESSIONS OF A REFORMED PERSONAL TRAINER

A SPECIAL PROGRAM—A SPECIAL GIFT

I HAD A RUNNING COACH when I lived back East. In the company of loping dogs, we propelled our bodies along dusty New England dirt roads. We pushed up endless hills and tightened back against perilous descents. Through peaceful pastures of munching cows and around the high school track teaming with young, agile students, we ran. In the summer, before a long run, we would set out jugs of water along the grueling, steamy route; one at the stop sign on the corner of Bucks Hill and Waterbury Road, and one against the last fencepost on Lahey's property where Amelia, the Lahey's black and white goat, feasted on clover and ignored our panting. In icy, treacherous winters we ran behind snow plows and slid on the slushy roads that were barely visible through whirling flakes and frozen eyelashes. If I cried in despair over aching lungs, my coach would turn around (running backwards in front of me) and encourage me to feel superior to everyone who drove by in an automobile. If I whined over throbbing muscles, he'd tell me to "tough it out." On one long trek, when I announced that I was nauseous, he advised me to stop just long enough to throw up and get back to the route. By the time I became a certified personal trainer, I was running six miles a day and pumping iron three days a week. I was a forty-five-year-old exercise fanatic.

There was no end to the stream of people who came to my workout studio wanting tight butts, flat abs, and slender legs. Women strove for the model's figure, men a weight lifters bulk.

They paid me well, and I trained them hard. Like my old running coach, I asked nothing of my clients that I didn't ask of myself. We walked, ran, and cycled together. We groaned through weightlifting and moaned into our stretches, and they remained committed, motivated by my disciplined system and observable results. Although I had packed on a few extra pounds in my late thirties, I had always been athletic. With the serious training, I had become lean, tight, youthful-looking, and smug. When a casual acquaintance asked when I'd be retiring my jogging shoes and passing my heavy weights on to the grandchildren, I huffed indignantly. "I'll run six miles a day and power lift forever. You don't retire from fitness." I was certain I had cornered the market on successful aging.

In 1996, I moved to the Pacific Northwest—to a rural little spot on the end of a peninsula. Soaring eagles and the snow-capped Cascade Mountains were magnificent sights from my window. I ran on the beach in the company of whales, started writing my first book, and got a job in the new wellness department of the local hospital. The position was a Phase III maintenance program personal trainer. I would be working with staff nurses to exercise and educate cardiac, diabetes, and COPD outpatients. The job was a good fit. In addition to my fitness business, I had worked in Connecticut as a medical assistant for fifteen years. But although I was no longer teaching and coaching die-hard fitness enthusiasts, in my personal life I continued to follow the narrow path of invincible athlete, keeping true to my belief that in the absence of chronic illness, extreme conditioning was beneficial. And I kept up the manic pace until being a wellness personal trainer unraveled the dogma and unveiled a broader vista. An old proverb says, "I never ask God to give me anything; I only ask him to put me where things are." I not only hadn't asked for anything, I hadn't asked for any particular placement, but I *had* landed in a setting that would offer exceptional "things."

The wellness clients were in various stages of rehabilitation. Some were weak after a cardiac event, others learning new breathing techniques, and some still reeling from a diabetes diagnosis. No one was planning to run a marathon or hoist mega-weights.

There was little interest in sculpting runway bodies or bulging biceps. Their goals were basic—stay alive, stay independent and active, and focus on optimal health.

My hovering was immediate. I patrolled the gym like a chaperone at a fifties sock hop. Strained hearts, weak lungs, and out-of-whack endocrine glands compromised my exercisers, keeping me on my toes and on the lookout for problems. Pulses were checked, blood pressures taken, oxygen saturations watched. If a cardiac client scratched a shoulder in mid-workout, I wanted to know if he was experiencing chest pain. When a pulmonary participant slowed his treadmill pace, I looked for shortness of breath. If a diabetic said she felt "funny," I insisted on a definition of "funny" and had her check her glucose. In the interest of safety and good patient care, my dialogue with them was constant.

Clients were also eager for conversation with fellow classmates. They shared medical histories, family dynamics, and the emotional ups and downs that came with their new health status. Folks who had lived on the peninsula most of their lives expounded on the old lay of the land, and newcomers talked about what had lured them to the area. Exotic vacation tales were offered, and new grand babies were announced. Over time, each class developed a unique personality. One morning group started discussing books and movies and brought in articles on medical advances for their maladies. In another class, the women talked recipes and gardens and the men sports. And one afternoon group raucously prattled on in hot debate about almost anything. For an hour a day, three days a week, exercisers in my six classes enjoyed their workout, and each other, while I monitored their vitals, taught them proper exercise techniques, and quizzed them for any health changes. As the days turned into weeks, and the weeks into months, clients got stronger, and I began to notice changes in myself.

Observing a cardiac patient just weeks out of surgery plodding one slow foot in front of the other on the treadmill, I questioned the sanity of wanting to outrun my last run. Listening to the click, click of an oxygen tank sending rhythmic bursts of air to a COPD sufferer pedaling a stationary bicycle one more minute, I wondered why I wasn't grateful for every easy inhale and exhale that I enjoyed. When a diet-conscious diabetic was jubilant over a glucose reading that bordered on normal, I realized how little I appreciated my freedom to enjoy a donut. Briefly, I contemplated the notion that with all the miles I had run in the name of fitness, when it came to inner improvement I had been running in place. Briefly, I considered I had been running to own a modicum of control, but the discomfort of those possibilities sent me fleeing back to my athlete's attitude. Pushing my body made me strong, physical prowess equated to a cut above, discipline created all the improvement I needed. The association with my clients served only to reinforce my desire for continued physical excellence. And then, like the proverb, "I never ask God to give me anything; I only ask him to put me where things are," the situation of wellness offered up one of those exceptional "things."

He was one hundred years old. Born in a sod house on the Nebraska prairie, he had formed a band at the same time Lawrence Welk was getting started. I met him when he joined one of my groups in the hospital program. His name was Jake. He was small and frail, his pulse was close to impossible to detect, and his blood pressure was quite low. He wobbled some getting up from the chair, leaning with both hands on his walker for support. With Jake, my hovering took on new proportions. On his first day in class, I linked an arm through his and applied a death grip to the underside of his forearm. Jake smiled and patted my other hand that was tightly attached to his upper arm, and we shuffled toward a bike. I adjusted the seat, helped him climb on, and secured his feet on the pedals and hands on the bars. He pushed one foot down and the pedals and handlebars began a slow rotation. His leg and arm muscles quivered. I stepped closer. His body stabilized and he pedaled a little harder. I was worried. What if a foot slipped off the pedal and he fell? What if he passed out? What if his hundred-year-old heart just quit, right there on the bike?

"Tell me how you're feeling, Jake," I asked in an insistent voice.

He grinned and pedaled faster.

"How hard do you feel you're working?" I quizzed.

He winked, raised both thumbs up and began to sing.

"On the road again ... Just can't wait to get on the road again."

The class howled with delight, and Jake continued on with his Willie Nelson tune. I sniveled through a mix of laughter and tears, and by the time my playful centenarian stopped singing, the understanding that successful aging was not about physical superiority was part of my heart.

The Jake encounter changed my focus. I tuned-in to the psyches of my eighty and ninety-year-old exercisers. They were happy. No matter the health issues, no matter the detours in the road, they all had a positive, upbeat outlook on life. Not driven by tomorrow, they appreciated today. With undaunted spirit and devilish humor, their countenance supported a longevity attitude. One ninety-plus gentleman, who always wore a tie to class, often said how fortunate he felt to live his life in such a beautiful environment. A ninety-year-old woman, who had moved to the peninsula to be closer to her daughter, said she had many old friends in California, but sure liked her new bridge partners. The same woman also scolded me when I shadowed her every move.

"You're just like my daughter, the two of you, constantly hovering instead of enjoying."

And then there was eighty-nine-year-old Lilly. Most days, before her wellness class, she'd be on the beach exercising her three Boston terriers. I was about to go for a run one morning when I saw her. I watched the dogs romp ahead and Lilly anchor the tip of her cane here and there as she glided through the sand and over driftwood. She stopped now and then, and the dogs would gather around her. Lilly addressed each pup by name,

"Aren't you the cutest girl, my Rosie."

Smiling, she looked across the blue-green bay at the majestic mountains, her eyes taking in the beauty as if for the first time. Her ruddy cheeks glowed in the early sun, the easy flow of her carriage evident of an inner order. The serenity of the woman was palpable. The run forfeited, I sat cross-legged in the sand. The beauty of aging with dignity and joy was evident in Lilly and all of my tranquil older exercisers. In that moment, I knew no matter the heft of the weights I lifted or the distance in miles I ran, a fruitful, loving maturity required looking within. As a wellness trainer I received a goodly supply of kudos from my cardiac, diabetes, and COPD people, but my older exercisers contributed the most valuable legacy. They cracked a fitness nut. In the company of extraordinary dispositions I saw gladness and contentment as components to a healthy lifestyle and graciousness, not glory, a hallmark of successful aging.

It was around this time that my ambition for running vanished. I had known for a while that the extreme exercise had been a transport away from many things in my life. Now, through my wellness clients, I saw that I was also running for the outward show, and I hadn't *run* into any significant personal development. So, I started to walk, an hour every day—up on the bluff high above the sea where pines were so thick in spots the sky disappeared, down to the water's edge where seagulls nestled in grains of sun-baked sand, around thick blackberry brambles in the dense woods. I felt a new kind of vigor, as much from the beauty as from the activity. In the absence of bettering my last run, I felt at peace. In the absence of pounding the pathways, my back stopped hurting and my knees didn't creak. Practicing what I preached to my exercisers, I focused on health rather than looks, inside fine-tuning instead of outside repair, but as can happen with all good intentions, a glitch in the road tampered with sensibility.

It was long, sleek, and silky. The soft rayon cascaded from the clips of the hanger like fall leaves drifting from tree limbs. The delicate print was black, brown, and white paisley. The top had a narrow cut that hugged close to the abdomen and hips. The tulip flare of the calf-length hemline added a sexy bounce. It was my favorite skirt. I was posed in front of the full-length mirror in the bedroom holding the skirt, still clipped to the hanger, against my body. Between working on the house and my wellness job, I hadn't worn anything feminine in a year, but on this particular day, I decided to dress up for lunch with an old college friend.

The skirt rippled down the middle of me like a thin scarf. Taking it off the hanger, I tossed the garment over my head and wiggled my torso through the forgiving elastic waistband, anticipating its sensual slide down my body. Instead, there was a pinching squeeze above my navel where the skirt was bunched like a strained rubber band. I unwound the material an inch or two, tugged at the hem, and gyrated my hips in an attempt to get things moved into place. The cat, awakened by the commotion, wove between my legs. I tripped over her, gracefully, and plopped to the floor, the skirt grabbing my middle like an old fashioned bellyband. I landed directly in front of the full-length mirror, bulges oozing over and around the size six A-line.

My mind raced. My favorite skirt!! How did I let this happen? Look at me—the hell with tranquility and inner peace. I'd start my old routine that very day. I'd run six miles, eat no more than fifteen hundred calories, get back to lifting ten pound weights. And then I heard the song on the radio. "On the road again ... Just can't wait to get on the road again." At first I laughed, recalling old Jake's comedic rendition of Willie, but the chortling turned quickly to me. I was quite a sight in a heap on the floor, the cat in the tangle of skirt in my lap. Then I wanted to cry. I was dismayed to find my old fanatical convictions so close to the surface, but the fretting abated when I remembered a conversation a few weeks back with Helen, a warm and cheerful seventy-year-old cardiac wellness client. We had talked about my upcoming lunch date. I mentioned wanting to wear my old skirt. Helen had advised against it. "I never keep any wearing apparel for more than three years," she said. "I'm forever evolving. I can't put yesterday's clothes on today's woman." I untangled myself from skirt and cat, slid comfortably into size twelve jeans and headed for lunch.

That evening I thought about Helen's words. Growing well-rounded in every sense, I didn't want to put yesterday's clothes on today's woman. The fit would be all wrong. I, too, was evolving—at a snail's pace—toward benevolent aging. I thought about all of my exercisers and my decision to accept the wellness job, and I attributed my meager successes in part to the proverb of asking to be put where "things" are. I believed my subconscious made that request of God on my behalf to place me in the loving presence of good people who had walked the path before me.

My clients, young and old, gave me many gifts. Their determination in the face of illness, strength in the presence of fear, and enduring spirit in the confusion of change contributed greatly to my personal growth. Association with my students was as much one of receiving

as of giving. My wish for all present and future champions pursuing the higher path to health is that you enjoy a successful passage
to wholeness in the surety of a wellness program. "No camel route
is long with good company."

13

QUESTIONS AND CONCERNS

What is the best way to get into Phase II Wellness if I haven't been hospitalized?

Physicians often prescribe a wellness program for their cardiac, diabetes, and pulmonary patients who are appropriate for the program, even without a recent hospitalization. If yours doesn't, you can ask him/her about a referral, or you can phone your local wellness department directly.

What should I bring to my Phase II diabetes intake interview?

If you have received a questionnaire (may be called a "D-Smart") prior to your intake interview, fill it out completely, and bring it with you to your appointment. The questionnaire helps the staff measure outcomes and encourages you to think about what changes you are ready to make. Also, bring a list of all medications you are currently taking, including prescription, over-the-counter, and herbal therapies, as well as your blood glucose monitoring equipment. Have your husband, wife, significant other, a friend, or a family member go to the appointment with you. They can help you answer and ask questions more thoroughly and be an extra set of ears when listening to the diabetes rehab coordinator. Bring your insurance information.

Are there any specific questions I should ask during my diabetes intake interview?

Questions will depend on where you are in the course of the disease. Always address the things you are most worried about as a diabetes patient. Ask about the cause of diabetes, how you can control it, how you should eat, and what resources are available to help you deal with the emotional impact of the disease. Also, ask to be shown how to properly use your blood glucose monitoring equipment, and find out what range your blood glucose numbers should fall into. Ask about length of program, cost, and schedule of Phase II diabetes payments particular to your insurance plan.

What should I bring to my Phase II cardiac intake interview?

Bring a list of your current medications, including prescription, over-the-counter, and herbal therapies. Bring a list of the goals you would like to accomplish in cardiac rehab. Have your husband, wife, significant other, a friend, or a family member go to the appointment with you. They can help you answer and ask questions more thoroughly and be an extra set of ears when listening to the cardiac rehab coordinator. Bring your insurance information.

Are there any specific questions I should ask during my cardiac intake interview?

Ask about the specific cardiac event that happened to you. Ask what you can expect to happen next regarding your condition. What's the prognosis? Ask your Phase II cardiac facilitator what goals they have for you and if the program is individualized for your particular needs. Ask about length of program, cost, and schedule of Phase II cardiac payments particular to your insurance plan.

What should I bring to my Phase II pulmonary intake interview?

A list of your medications, including prescription, over-the-counter, and herbal therapies. Bring a health history and a list of any questions, especially your concerns about exercising with COPD. Have your husband, wife, significant other, a friend, or a family member go to the appointment with you. They can help you answer and ask questions more thoroughly and be an extra set of ears when listening to the pulmonary rehab coordinator. Bring your insurance information.

Are there any specific questions I should ask during my pulmonary intake interview?

Address whatever issues you may have regarding your illness. Ask questions about your specific pulmonary diagnosis. Ask about length of program, cost, and schedule of Phase II pulmonary payments particular to your insurance plan.

Will my insurance pay for Phase II diabetes, cardiac, pulmonary classes?

Since insurance payments can be regionally dependent and often vary from plan to plan, a schedule of payments approved by your insurance carrier (including Medicare and supplemental) will be discussed during your intake interview.

Does any insurance pay for Phase III maintenance exercise?

Medicare does not pay for Phase III maintenance, and most other insurance plans do not pay. There are, however, a few that do, so it never hurts to check with your insurance carrier.

What should I wear to my exercise class?

Wear loose, comfortable clothing. If you wear a sweatshirt or sweater, have a tee shirt underneath so the top layer can be removed in case you get too warm. Elastic-waist sweatpants or slacks are ideal. Some folks are most comfortable in shorts. Sturdy, supportive shoes with backs and rubber soles are a must for comfort and safety. No sandals, high heels, flip-flops, or slip-ons.

What should I bring to exercise class? What about water and a towel?

Bring as little as possible. Some exercisers like to have a small towel with them for excess perspiration. You can bring your own water, but there will be water coolers or drinking fountains in or near the gym. If you're diabetic and regularly check your glucose, bring glucose monitoring equipment. Diabetics should also have a snack or juice with them.

Will I be able to change my clothes after exercise?

Yes. Although most hospital wellness facilities do not have locker rooms or showers, they do have restrooms.

Should I eat right before my class?

Have something to eat about an hour before exercise. Exercising immediately after eating can cause nausea. Exercising on an empty stomach can cause dizziness, lightheadedness, and for some diabetics a dangerous drop in blood glucose levels. Also, diabetics are advised to bring a light snack or juice to class to manage the general possibility of low blood glucose during and after exercise.

What should I do if I can't make a class?

Call and let the staff know you'll be absent, particularly if you are ill. The wellness staff will be interested in any health changes and may have some helpful information or advice to offer.

I'm in a structured maintenance program with assigned classes. Will I ever be able to change my class time?

If there are openings in other classes, the staff will do their best to accommodate you.

Can I stay in the maintenance program forever?

Yes. Sometimes other health issues come up that disrupt an exercise schedule, but the staff will work to get you back into maintenance when you are medically released to exercise. You may start again with a different or lighter workout than the one you were doing before the onset of the new illness.

Once I'm assigned to a structured maintenance class, will I lose my spot if I go away on vacation?

Every wellness program will have its own vacation policy. In general, class place is not lost because of a few weeks vacation. If you plan on an extended absence, you may be taken off the class roster and your name put on a waiting list. You can call the staff when you return and discuss re-entry. Depending on enrollment, it may not be possible to return to your old class time.

Can I get back into maintenance if I'm out for an extended period with an illness or surgery?

Again, every wellness program will have its own policy, but participants are usually welcome to return to the program after an extended illness. You will need a medical release from your doctor and possibly a new exercise prescription. If you were in a structured class, it may not be possible to return to your old class time.

I can never find my pulse, and my hands are too shaky for me to fill out an exercise log. How will I manage by myself if I have to do those things in my maintenance class?

You are never by yourself in wellness maintenance. The staff will encourage as much independence as possible, but they are also available to work with you when help is needed. If necessary, the nurse or trainer will take your pulse and post your vitals and workout on your exercise log. Many programs are computerized, eliminating posting workouts by hand.

If regular participation in maintenance exercise keeps my blood pressure and blood glucose numbers in a good range, can I stop taking my medications?

It can be dangerous to abruptly stop taking certain medications. Even with numbers consistently within normal limits, you should never discontinue any medication without first consulting with your doctor.

In my maintenance program, blood pressures are usually taken once a week. Since my stroke I worry about my numbers. Can I have my blood pressure checked more frequently?

In general, a once-a-week blood pressure check is sufficient, but the schedule is not carved in stone. There will be clients who have pressures checked every time they come to class, as well as those checked once-a-week who occasionally request an additional reading. Also, in cases where there have been fluctuations in blood pressures or medications have been changed, the wellness staff may start checking those folks more frequently for a while. There will also be times when staff will check a client's blood pressure during a workout.

If a friend or family member comes to exercise class with me, can they exercise too?

No. Only registered clients are cleared to use the exercise equipment.

I look after my granddaughter. Can she come to class with me?

It's fine if she's old enough to adhere to gym safety rules and is willing to entertain herself with quiet activities, such as reading or coloring. It's not advisable to bring toddlers to class.

My Labrador retriever is a therapy dog. She goes everywhere with me. Can I bring her to class?

Therapy and Seeing Eye dogs can accompany their owners to exercise classes. Clients with therapy dogs may be asked to present a doctor's written prescription for the animal. One sticky wicket is the possibility of another exerciser in your group having an allergy to dogs. Changing classes can solve the problem. In most cases, the wellness staff will find constructive canine solutions.

Even though physically I am able to use a lot of the machines, I really like the treadmill best. Can I stay on it for the whole class time?

If you are able to use a variety of equipment, it is advisable to do so. Cross training is good for your body. If your class is large, the program may have a time limit rule on equipment. For example, fifteen minutes per person per machine is common. This ensures that everyone has a chance to use different equipment. But even in programs that do have a time limit rule, there can be exceptions. Perhaps a medical condition limits a wellness exerciser to one specific machine. If the class is small on a particular day, the time limit rule may be waived.

I wasn't allowed to use the treadmill one day because I was wearing flip-flops. It was only that one time, and I felt the staff should have made an exception.

Be grateful. The staff should never make exceptions where client safety is concerned.

I love my exercise maintenance class, but sometime the music others select to play during our workout is awful. What can I do?

There should be ample opportunity for everyone to have a shot at selecting the music, which can mean that on some days some people may not be thrilled with the tunes. If you're really unhappy with the music on a particular day, you can always suggest an alternative CD or radio station. Or you can get in the habit of bringing a portable player with earphones to class so you can plug into music of your liking. Sometimes class discussions replace music. Perhaps you can get the ball rolling with a timely topic. Differences make life interesting, if not always enjoyable.

There are a variety of personalities, temperaments, health issues, and life stories in wellness exercise classes. To maintain a good perspective, remember:

1. It has been a tough road for all of you.
2. You're all doing the best you can.
3. Every moment of every day, the choice to initiate good feelings and positive outcomes is an available option.

14

FINDING A WELLNESS PROGRAM

THERE ARE A FEW WAYS to locate a hospital wellness program in your area. You can start by calling the nearest hospital and asking if they have one. If they do not run a program of their own, they may be able to refer you to one that is reasonably close to home. Another avenue is to check with the nurse in your primary care physician's office, or your specialist's office. Your local library can also be a good resource.

If you have access to a computer and the Internet, go to a search engine (google, for example) and type:
"Cardiac rehabilitation" and the name of your state
"Pulmonary rehabilitation" and the name of your state
"Diabetes wellness programs" and the name of your state

You can contact state and local chapters of the American Heart Association, American Diabetes Association, or American Lung Association.

For general information and pamphlets specific to your illness and exercise:

American Diabetes Association
1701 North Beauregard Street
Alexandria, VA 22311
Phone: 1-800-342-2383
Internet: www.diabetes.org

American Heart Association
7272 Greenville Avenue
Dallas, TX 75231-4596
Phone: 1-800-242-8721
Internet: www.americanheart.org

American Lung Association
61 Broadway, 6th Floor
New York, NY 10006
Phone: (212) 315-8700 or 1-800-LUNGUSA for nearest
lung association
Internet: www.lungusa.org

GLOSSARY

Aerobic exercise: Exercise in which sufficient oxygen is continually supplied to the body.

Anaerobic exercise: Exercise that creates an oxygen deficit.

Aortic valve: A heart value between the left ventricle and the aorta.

Cardiovascular disease: Any one of numerous dysfunctions of the heart and blood vessels.

Chronic obstructive pulmonary disease (COPD): A group of lung conditions, such as, emphysema, chronic bronchitis, and asthma, characterized by diminished lung function.

Claudication: Leg weakness and cramping calf pain caused by poor blood circulation to the leg muscles.

Diabetes mellitus: A disorder of carbohydrate, protein, and fat metabolism characterized by insufficient (or no) insulin secretion or utilization.

Flexibility: Joint range of motion determined by muscle, tendon, and ligament length.

Glucose: A simple sugar found in some foods, especially fruits. A source of energy occurring in human and animal body fluids.

Insulin: A hormone secreted by beta cells in the pancreas in response to increased glucose in the blood. Insulin regulates the metabolism of glucose and the processes for metabolism of proteins, fats, and carbohydrates.

Isometric resistance exercise: Muscular tension against an immovable object.

Isotonic exercise: Exercising against a movable resistance.

Pulmonary function tests: A measure of how well lungs take in and release air, and how efficiently oxygen is transferred into the blood.

Nephropathy: Any disorder of the kidney.

Neuropathy: Inflammation and degeneration of the peripheral nerves.

Pulse oximeter: A devise used to detect the percentage of hemoglobin that is saturated with oxygen.

Retinopathy: An eye disorder caused by changes in the retinal blood vessels.

Telemetry: The transmission of heart rhythm to a receiving station.

Treadmill stress test: A walk test, on a motorized treadmill, that records heart rate and rhythm during exercise. Electrodes are attached to chest, speed and incline are gradually increased, and a doctor monitors heart activity. Time on the treadmill is determined by level of conditioning and recovery.

BIBLIOGRAPHY

Cooper, Kenneth H. *Aerobics*. New York, New York: Bantam Books, 1968.

Cotton, Richard T., ed. *Exercise for Older Adults*. San Diego, CA: American Council on Exercise, 1998.

Glanze, Walter D., ed. *Mosby's Medical Dictionary, 3rd edition*. St. Louis, MO: The C.V. Mosby Company, 1990.

Hales, Dianne. *An Invitation to Health, 6th edition*. Redwood City, CA: The Benjamin/Cummings Publishing Co., Inc., 1994.

Hill, Napoleon and Michael J. Ritt, Jr. *Keys to Positive Thinking*. New York: Plume, 1999.

Kolata, Gina. *Ultimate Fitness The Quest for Truth About Exercise and Health*. New York: Farrar, Straus and Giroux, 2003.

Kübler-Ross, Elisabeth. *The Wheel of Life*. New York: Scribner, 1997.

Magill's Medical Guide: Health and Illness, Vol. l. CA: Salem Press, Inc., 1995.

Moll, Louise B. *The World's Greatest Cryptograms*. New York: Paschal, Barbara. Balance Aerobics. P.O. Box 4123, Sequim, WA: 2003. Sterling Publishing Company, Inc. For Quality Paperback Book Club, 1997.

Rakel, Robert E. MD, ed. *Conn's Current Therapy*. Philadelphia, PA: W.B. Saunders Company, 1999.

Robertson, Loarn, acquisitions ed. *Guidelines for Cardiac Rehabilitation and Secondary Prevention Programs, Third Edition.* American Association of Cardiovascular & Pulmonary Rehabilitation. Champaign, Ill: Human Kinetics, 1999.

Sharkey, Brian J. *Fitness and Health*, 4th edition. Champaign, IL: Human Kinetics, 1997.

Williams, Melvin. *Lifetime Fitness and Wellness, 3rd edition.* Madison, WI: WCB Brown & Benchmark, 1993.

———⋙●⋘———

CONTRIBUTORS

Benner, Amber, B.S.N.

Burr, Jan, B.A., L.M.P.

Gentle, Frank, certified personal trainer, exercise technician

Hazard, Mitzi, P.T., C.D.E.

Holmes, Andrew G., tai chi chuan instructor

Lemons, Gary, certified yoga instructor, poet

Norwood, Frank

Paschal, Barbara, P.T.

Price, Mary, exercise physiologist

Riddle, Katherine, R.R.T.

Schmidt, Nancy, B.S.N.

Short, Holly, B.A.

Smith-Poling, Sandra, M.D., director for emergency medical
    services Jefferson County, commander 446 aeromedical staging
    squadron, McCord Air Force Base, Tacoma, WA

Stein, Jerry, B.S., J.D., L.L.M.

Vane, Barbara, certified personal trainer, exercise technician

Whitney, David S., M.D., board certified orthopedic surgeon

WELLNESS TITLES FROM CAVEAT PRESS

Glimmers: A Journey into Alzheimer's Disease
by Heidi Hamilton, Ph.D
ISBN: 1-883991-79-X / Paperback: $14.95

Kentro Body Balance: The Secret Pleasures of Posture
by Angelika Thusius
ISBN: 1-883991-0-0 / Paperback: $23.95

*One Trip Around the Sun: A Guide to Using Diet, Herbs, Exercise and
Meditation to Harmonize with the Seasons*
by Rory Lipsky, L.Ac.
ISBN: 1-883991-85-4 / Paperback: $19.95

Yin Yoga: Outline of a Quiet Practice
by Paul Grilley
ISBN: 1-883991-43-9 / Paperback: $15.95